MW00586439

Reaching Beyond

Virginia Neary Carrithers

COPYRIGHT © 2017 VIRGINIA TICE NEARY CARRITHERS
All rights reserved.

No part of this publication may be reproduced or transmitted in any form or by any means, mechanical or electronic, including photocopying and recording, or by any information storage and retrieval system, without permission in writing from the author or publisher (except by a reviewer, who may quote brief passages and/or short, brief video clips in a review.)

For permission requests, write to the publisher, addressed "Attention: Permissions Coordinator," at the address below.

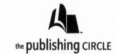

the **publishing** CIRCLE

admin@ThePublishingCircle.com

or

THE PUBLISHING CIRCLE, LLC
Regarding: Virginia Tice Neary Carrithers
1603 Capitol Avenue
Suite 310
Cheyenne, Wyoming 82001

The publisher is not responsible for the author's website, other mentioned websites, dead or expired links to any website, redirected links, or content of any website that is not owned by the publisher.

All content is the author's opinion only.

REACHING BEYOND:
ONE WOMAN'S INSPIRING & UNCOMPROMISING WILL TO LIVE
THROUGH LOVE & LOSS WITH MULTIPLE SCLEROSIS

FIRST EDITION
ISBN 978-1-947398-03-0 (pbk)

Cover design & book interior design by Michele Uplinger

DEDICATION

I dedicate this book
to my brother,
William Arnold Tice, Jr.,
a brave man
who lived as a quadriplegic
from the age of 21, when he broke his neck,
to the age of 55, when he died of cancer.

CONTENTS

FOREWORD

ON DECEMBER 14, 2016, ON A GREY, rainy Pacific Northwest day,
I received an email from *The Caretaker Gazette* with this newly posted
advertisement:

ARGENTINA PATAGONIA
FRONTIER CALLING!

Artist's assistant and companion needed
in the Andes of Northern Patagonia for a
determined woman with Multiple Sclerosis.
I need a commitment of a minimum of one
month, the longer the better. I am an artist and
an experienced horsewoman. I believe in the
healing power of creativity, as well as the love of
nature and her creatures. My ranch is located
in a non-touristic part of beautiful Patagonia,
nestled in the foothills of the Andes, in the
heart of the real Gaucho culture. In the winter
months (May through November) we may be
changing locations. I will pay all expenses
when together. This is not a salaried position,
as it is a volunteer opportunity. In exchange for
adventure, fun, basic food and housing, you
will be my co-creator in art projects. Duties
include, but are not limited to, help with the
horses. Important that we enjoy each other's
company. Free time to be arranged as needed
and wanted. You should have a mastery of
English, Spanish a major plus, good computer

skills, a driver's license, and the ability to drive a manual/stick-shift. Please send a description of why you are interested, résumé if you have one, something about yourself, your age and a photo to Patagoniapearl@gmail.com Please see my webpage at www.creativityheals.org. Thank you for your interest. I look forward to sharing with you.

I ticked off every requirement except for Spanish. I have enough Spanish to locate the bathroom and feed myself, so I figured that should be enough and immediately sent off a reply:

Dear Ginny,

I just received your advertisement for an artist's assistant and companion from *The Caretaker Gazette*. When I read your requirements, and reviewed your website, I knew I had to apply. I am inspired by the fact that you've lived with MS gracefully for 40 years, and in all the setbacks of living with chronic illness, have forged a course forward combining creativity with your love of nature and animals. A large part of this opportunity's appeal is that you are a creative and, of course, the horses.

Also appealing is the opportunity to return to Argentina. About ten years ago, I met up with a friend living in Buenos Aires and we traveled throughout the country for three weeks. I fell in love with the landscape, people and culture and have been longing to return and immerse in Argentina's inspiration.

I believe in the power of creativity and nature to heal. Three years ago, I closed my personal training business after the deaths of a dear friend, my mother, and mother-in-law. I was broken and needed time to reconnect. When I sat down in front of a blank page after a twelve-year writing hiatus, my grief was so deep that I couldn't string together an entire sentence. With no defenses or filters left, I took dictation, jotting down the few words that came.

In the spring of 2014, I asked a writer friend what I should do with the mess of words accumulating at an alarming rate. I thought they might be poems, but wasn't sure. I was a prose writer. Her sage advice—find a poetry class. I found a beginning workshop and, through that, a mentor. In March of 2015, I attended the Tucson Festival of Books as winner of the poetry contest. To say the conference was life-changing sounds cliché, but it was. It affirmed me as a poet and gave credence to my voice. What I have to say matters.

I am currently engaged in December's Tupelo Press 30/30 Project. I've committed to writing a poem a day for thirty days in an effort to raise money for Tupelo Press—a non-profit, independent press providing a platform for emerging voices, culturally specific communities, and literary art forms not fostered by mainstream publishers. I've also been nominated for a 2017 Pushcart Prize for my prose piece, *Bone of the Past*.

My voice and appreciation for other cultures were further strengthened on a sojourn to Thailand from May-October of 2015. I taught English as a second language in a government school to middle and high school students in rural Amnat Charoen Province in eastern Thailand. I had 430 student contact hours/week (no that's not a typo) and continued to write in every spare moment, creating an email blog called *The Thai Diaries*.

I have given myself the gift of this year to pursue my writing and all activities, including travel, that inform it. I have been house-sitting to keep a roof over my head and have also had a month-long artist's residency. House sitting has given me time and space to write.

Spiritually, I was raised Catholic, but subscribe to Buddhism and have had a morning meditation practice for the past two years. Meditation keeps me grounded in, and appreciative of, the present moment. Really, it's all we have.

As per your ad: I am 58 and in good health and physical condition. I walk two to four miles most days and am an avid hiker and yoga practitioner. I have decent computer skills and am adept with a stick shift after a bit of practice.

I am an experienced horsewoman and am very comfortable in a farm/ranch setting, having grown up on rural Kauai with dogs, cats, chickens, pigs, birds and a horse. As mentioned earlier, I was a personal trainer by trade, specializing in corrective exercise and sought-after for my skills with special populations. Over the course of seven years, I worked with clients with Parkinson's and MS, helping them to maintain as much stability, balance, mobility, and muscle as possible.

I am willing to commit for an initial period of three-months. Given that the situation is a good fit for both of us, I'd be open to discussing a further extension. It is my sincere hope that we'll be able to speak further about this exciting opportunity. I am curious as to what being a co-creator in your art projects and universe entails!

With warm regards,

Burky Achilles

In further correspondence, I learned Ginny wanted me to ghostwrite her memoirs. As a traveling writer in need of a roof and a project, I said yes.

On February 14, 2017, after a four-hour, $300 USD taxi ride from the nearest airport in Neuquén, first on paved, then gravel roads, I arrived at Ginny's dusty chacra just outside the tiny Cowtown of El Heucú. After reviewing over 350 pages of timelines written with previous volunteers over the course of two-years from 2009-2010, spanning Ginny's birth through 2010, along with various media articles from the 1970s through the 1990s, Ginny's journals and her artwork, I sat down in my ranchita, thirty yards from the cacophony of the main house, and began to write.

Burky Achilles

APRIL 30, 2017

Reaching Beyond

WATERLOO

CRYSTAL ISLAND RANCH

LOUISVILLE

NEW YORK

NEW ORLEANS

Reaching
Beyond

ARGENTINA

BUENOS AIRES

EL HUECÚ

EL HEUCÚ, NORTHERN PATAGONIA, ARGENTINA

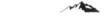

FEBRUARY 21, 2017

MY EYES ARE FAILING AND IT'S painful for me to focus on any kind of screen or text, so my current volunteer is typing this for me. I've spent the past few weeks with a patch over my right eye and dark glasses over that to keep out any light. My back is also quite painful. I broke my L1 vertebrae in a fall in 2009 and while my rehab went well throughout 2010, the combination of a newly recurring bout of Multiple Sclerosis and the subsequent weakness in my spine leave me in quite a bit of pain. I can sit in my wheelchair for no more than three hours at a time, then I must be helped into bed to lie down to ease my back.

The situation here is difficult. My main caregiver, Rosa, quit last night and says this time (she quits one to two times a month) she means it. She has some intestinal health issues and is in pain herself. Despite having been hospitalized over the weekend, she was back at work Monday morning and is doing a thirty-six-hour shift. Typically, she and her sister, Monica, alternate twelve-hour shifts with Rosa assisting me days and Monica working nights. Claudia is my caregiver on weekends. She comes Friday evening and is here through Sunday evening when Monica returns.

I'm fighting hard to keep a positive attitude, but at times I am discouraged by the pain, and seeming futility of my plight as well as the constant worry over money and employees needed to attend me and run this place. There are six people who work here part or full-time and while I speak some Spanish, it's a mish-mash and grammatically abhorrent. You'd think I'd be fluent after thirty-plus years living in Argentina. Maybe the brain lesions, a marker of my MS, are affecting my language center. My speech slurs too, but that could be a function of the quarter of a pain pill I take for my back or the fatigue of chronic illness or both. Who knows? Anyway, trying to make myself understood in my adopted language is difficult and draining.

While my life is rich in tender-loving care, I have no income. At nearly 68, my "retirement" is dependent on the sale of a home and barn on two-and-a-half acres in Colorado. I also own this twenty-acre chacra in El Heucú in Northern Patagonia. Thank God for Sky. Without her, my world as I know it would cease to spin.

Sky, my cherished twenty-eight-year-old daughter, whose long blond braid swings down her strong back, rides the cordillera as well as any man. With her working dogs serving as guardians, she surveys the 100,000-acre Estancia Ranquilco entrusted to her. Blue eyes laugh with the joy of the land, and the cattle, sheep, and goats she raises and protects. Only five-feet tall, she is tiny, but oh so mighty. She manages the land with her partner, Chano, and her two-year-old son Leonides, or Leo (pronounced Lay-Oh) on her hip.

Sky lives an hour-and-a-half away in Buta Mallin and is coming Thursday afternoon for the night to help sort things out with Rosa. I'm sure Sky's arrival will give me a much-needed boost. In the past few years as I've become increasingly bed and wheelchair ridden, we have talked of moving me to San Martin de los Andes to a nursing facility. The burden of running the chacra and keeping me here is becoming too much for all concerned. It may be time.

But, oh, the chacra.

Originally, I never saw myself living here because it's under-stimulating in many ways, yet in other ways it's not. At the chacra I must go more within than I'm used to. I used to get outer stimulation. Now I have to go within for inner stimulation, which means my art. Once again, I've been running from my art and now I've completely lost my right hand, my drawing and painting hand, to paralysis. But I have a left hand, and if it can feed me, it can draw and paint too. It's indicative that I don't want to do my art, but I'm going to do it. I'm going to quit running and root deep like these Lombardi poplars. Maybe deeper. I don't know. What I do know is when Rosa laid me on my poncho on the grass yesterday and I looked up at the towering poplars swaying in the wind, dropping their golden leaves on my cheeks, it was like kisses from the sky. These trees are my inspiration. This chacra a grounding place. My daughter will always come back here because of the ranches: the Colopilli winter grounds, the Buta Mallin summer grounds, and Ranquilco.

These twenty acres just out of El Heucú, have their own rustic beauty, but even so, the land is a far cry from the glossy web depiction of Estancia Ranquilco with its river and 100,000 acres or my 3000-acre corner of it. A five-mile stretch of the trout-filled Trocoman River runs through the heart of the corner, named simply, Trocoman. Though really, while the Trocoman is mine on paper, I am too crippled to ride the three-hours in on horseback from Buta Mallin. The responsibility for Trocoman, as for so many things these days, has fallen to Sky.

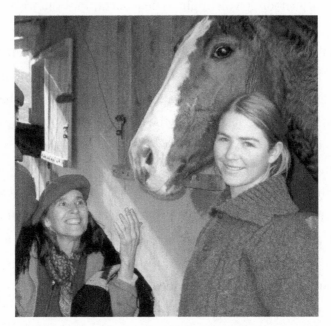

HERE I AM IN THE STABLES WITH HANDSOME
RUBIO ROYALE, A RACING QUARTER HORSE
STALLION, AND MY BEAUTIFUL DAUGHTER, SKY.
(EL HUECÚ, PATAGONIA, ARGENTINA, 2015)

NEW ORLEANS, LOUISIANA

1976

I WAS TWENTY-SEVEN AND COMING INTO my own as one of Louisiana's first female racehorse trainers. I'd earned my license in 1974 under the tutelage of a former jockey, Mr. Cleat—a slight, balding man with a big heart, gentle voice and velvet hands with the horses. He referred to me as "Sweet Ginny Lee" and always had time for my thousands of questions.

My debut as a racehorse trainer in 1973 was with Last Time Up at Evangeline Downs in Lafayette, Louisiana. This steel grey filly had been returned to Bob Levi's farm in Folsom because she couldn't win a race. She was sick and Bob wanted to sell her. Instead, I talked him into letting me nurse her back to health and trained her per Mr. Cleat's sound advice. We picked a short race to start—a quarter mile.

At Evangeline Downs, the horses were led into the gates, nickering, prancing, their energy high with the knowledge of what was coming.

At the bell, Last Time Up lurched from the gate and fell to her knees. I couldn't believe it. Evangeline Downs was not only my first race as a trainer, but Last Time Up was my boyfriend's horse. People were already skeptical of a female trainer. This was a disaster. However, when Bob nudged me and I opened my eyes, Last Time Up was on her feet and catching up to the field of horses far ahead of her. She was all heart and came in second in a photo finish.

I was on my way, but there were complications.

Bob Levi, my boyfriend and Last Time Up's owner, was one. I met Bob in the early 70s in a bar in the French Quarter on a night out with my sister, Sandra, and my fiancée, David Neary. Bob was ten years older, well-dressed and put-together, sexy in the way men with money often are. Money lends them an air of invincibility and, impervious to the worries of the world, they take what they want. That night, even though Bob knew I was with David, he made several passes that were hard to ignore.

After David and I married, Bob, who had a wife and two kids in the burbs, continued to pursue me by hooking up with my sister Sandra. Even though she knew he was married, Sandra couldn't resist Bob's suave charm and open wallet. What David and Sandra didn't know was that Bob was connected to the New Orleans' infamous mafia through his best friend, who happened to be the mob's lawyer. At that time, the mob owned all the best restaurants in the French Quarter and was heavily involved in horse racing. Bob always hedged his bets.

WATERLOO, IOWA

1965

DAVID NEARY WAS HANDSOME AND SEXY in a Midwest, clean-cut, track star, football quarterback kind of way. An Iowa boy, we had a history. We had been together since I was seventeen. He was nineteen and in college at nearby University of Northern Iowa. David and I met when my friend Janice and I were out on one of our many flirting expeditions to College Hill in my dad's Corvette Stingray. The older men appealed to us as the high school boys were pimply and immature. They loved Janice and me almost as fervently as the high school girls loved to hate us.

Sister Sandra, five years older than me, was partially responsible for that hatred. The summer I was fifteen, Dad sent me to visit Sandra in New Orleans where she attended Sophie Newcomb College at Tulane University. Sandra introduced me to the three b's—bras, boys and bars. She cut my hair, plucked my eyebrows and handed me a fake

I.D. Nature finished my transformation. As we were constantly at the pool by day, my dark-blonde hair developed golden-blonde highlights, while my flat chest developed into a 32D. The little baby fat left at waist and cheeks and the backs of my arms seemed to melt in those first weeks of southern heat.

I had never had a drink, nor did I know what "let's do it" meant, but at Bruno's Bar I learned to flirt—and loved it. Guys lined up for my number. I became known as a tease, but didn't care.

Although there were a couple of close calls, I had no intention of sleeping with any of these guys. I was bait and Sandra reeled in what she wanted and left the rest to flounder. The power of my new-found sexuality was intoxicating.

When I returned to Iowa at the end of summer, Janice hardly recognized me, but we fell in again easily enough, as we had been inseparable since grade school. Janice graciously let me take the lead on our social activities and I took that responsibility seriously. After the excitement of New Orleans, Iowa had become a place from which to escape. Janice and I would drive the Stingray to Lacrosse, Wisconsin to buy Coors beer with my fake I.D. We'd drive to Colorado to camp for the weekend. We'd drive to College Hill to flirt. No matter what, we drove, until I met David.

David and I dated throughout my senior year of high school. When I graduated in 1967 in the top one-percent of my class, I gravitated to Sophie Newcomb College at Tulane University like a moth to a porchlight, partly because Sandra still lived in New Orleans and partly because I had grown to love The Big Easy—the flash and sizzle, beignets and French roast in the mornings and beads and bourbon the nights leading up to Mardi Gras.

The freedom I had experienced in New Orleans with Sandra and during my own exploits in Iowa with Janice, then David, came to an abrupt halt at Sophie Newcomb. There was a ten o'clock curfew. I could only leave campus with a companion. They expected me to share a room with a stranger and bathrooms and showers with multiple strangers. As the weeks went on, I found myself pining for David back home in Waterloo. After a year and a half at Sophie Newcomb, I transferred to the University of Northern Iowa. It was January 1969 and David and I were together again.

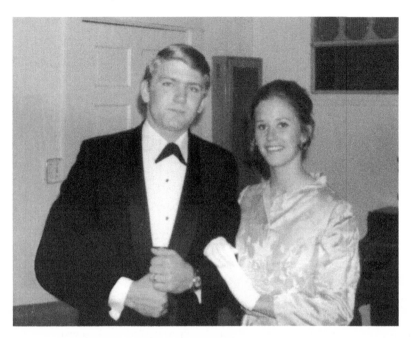

MY COLLEGE-AGED BOYFRIEND AND FUTURE HUSBAND, DAVID NEARY, AND ME POSING BEFORE MY HIGH SCHOOL PROM.
(WATERLOO, IOWA, 1967)

WATERLOO, IOWA

MARCH 1969

MARCH IN IOWA WAS A NOTHING SEASON. Dirty snow piled on the sides of the road, ice in the mornings and evenings, gravel on the roads that weren't already paved, and take your chances on the rest. My parents were wisely vacationing in the Grand Caymans, seemingly in love again, with Dad semi-retired from his psychiatry practice and writing poetry and short stories, and Mother, for the time being, stabilized.

Mother had had a nervous breakdown in 1958 when I was nine and Sandra and Bill were twelve and fourteen. Susie was four. Nobody said a word other than Dad who told us as we straggled in from outdoors one hot afternoon that Mother was going on a two-week vacation. Puzzled, we asked why mother would want to go on vacation without us. When, exactly, was she coming back? Our questions were ignored or deflected.

Two weeks passed into three, and our questioning became relentless. Finally, Dad broke under our siege and told us that no, Mother was not on vacation, but at Menninger's Mental Health Hospital in Topeka, Kansas. When my father dutifully piled us into the car to visit her a few months later, I refused to see her. Instead, I waited in the car. I could not help feeling that us kids had driven Mother away, leaving in her wake an efficient woman hired to cook and clean, starch and press, and little more.

I do not remember the day Mother left for Menninger's. None of my siblings do, either. What I remember is how radiant Mother appeared nine months later as she stepped from the cab and strolled up our front walk with her small suitcase in her white-gloved hand and patent leather purse in the crook of her arm. I remember how she stooped inside the front door with arms held wide to little Susie who flew into them, then how she stood with Susie in her arms and hugged Sandra and Bill in turn and how when it came to me, I ran upstairs to my room and hid under the bed. I wanted nothing to do with her.

So, here we were, eleven years later, in 1969, ready to celebrate my twentieth birthday. With Mother and Dad in Grand Cayman, David and I decided to drive to his family's place in Scranton, Iowa. Because it was early March and the weather was volatile, we commandeered Mother's big Lincoln Continental for the trip. It was like navigating an ocean tanker, but given the snow and ice, safer than the Stingray. Besides, the Stingray had a history. At 405 horsepower, 420 cubic inches and feather light, that big cat was dangerous. Janice and I had pushed it to 160 mph and laughed until it began to shake. Mother and Dad called it Hard Luck Harry, as on separate occasions both Mother and I had wrecked it.

Seated around the living room in Scranton, dinner and the dishes long done, David's parents had just wandered off to bed when the phone rang. It was my Uncle George. Brother Bill had wrecked Hard Luck Harry.

Later that night at the hospital in Waterloo, David and I found Bill lying in bed, a Stryker frame screwed to his skull. His injury was at C3, leaving him paralyzed from the neck down. He was able to talk a bit and move his eyes, but that was the extent of it. Susie was two doors down, having her appendix out, Sandra was on her way home from New Orleans and Mother and Dad were navigating their way back from Grand Cayman.

Bill, ever the intellectual and artist, had been home at Mother's and Dad's place for about three months. He had dropped out of the pre-med program at University of Iowa. Medical school had never been Bill's idea, but since junior high, while Bill was reveling in art classes and mechanics, Dad had been plotting Bill's course through med school. The pressure was ceaseless and when Bill arrived home unannounced after having invested over a year-and-a-half in the program, Dad retreated to his den and shut that door.

On the night of the accident, Bill had been home with his buddy Tim for the evening, along with their friend Jack Daniels and a tray full of ice. After a drink or four, they hopped into Hard Luck Harry for a little high-speed spin around town. On that moonless night, Bill never saw the patch of black ice or the cement upright at the railroad crossing. He slammed into the upright at over eighty miles per hour and his neck snapped. Tim walked away with a few bruises.

As I sat with Bill in the hospital that night, all I could think was that things would have been different had *I* taken Hard Luck Harry. Left with the Lincoln, Bill and Tim likely would not have gone out.

Given that I couldn't change the course of Bill's outcome, I took turns sitting vigil—first with David, then with Sandra and Mother and Dad as they showed up. Mother, curvaceously full- figured, but short at 5'2", seemed to have lost those precious two-inches. Somehow, she had folded in on herself between Grand Cayman and Bill's hospital room. Dad, never handsome at his best, had aged ten years, looking like the psychiatric patients he sometimes described as "unreachable."

Sandra, was of course, Sandra. She walked in as if she owned the place and immediately started interrogating the hospital staff and doctors as to Bill's prognosis.

Throughout Bill's first weeks in the hospital, I had lots of solo time to think. One morning the thought I might be pregnant settled over me. Maybe it was the nausea. It came out of nowhere, but with such certainty that I could not ignore it. Within a few days a doctor confirmed my suspicion.

By the end of March, I had found Doctor William Carlos in Kansas City. On a sunny morning in early April, I showered and dressed carefully in my Bonnie and Clyde suit and beret, then David and I took the train to Kansas City. We rode in silence. David and I had never really talked about it. Neither of us had words for what there was to say. Each in our own way just wanted this behind us.

At the station's curb, we paced. A half hour later, Doctor William Carlos arrived in his fluorescent green Cadillac convertible with white leather seats. After I handed over the cash, he drove us to his little office in the slums of Kansas City. I was three months along. There were no painkillers. I remember the tugging and pulling as Doctor William Carlos worked—sweat beading his brow. Were his lips pursed behind that surgical mask? I did not know. What I did know was it hurt like hell. But this pain was nothing compared to the day-in, day-out misery my parents faced over the loss of Bill's future and now how to manage and provide for their twenty-three-year-old son, given that he would remain a quadriplegic for the rest of his life.

WATERLOO, IOWA

SEPTEMBER 1969

AFTER A BRIEF STINT HOME IN JULY, Bill was sent to Yonkers Rehabilitation Center in Des Moines, Iowa. At 6'1" and 180 pounds of deadweight, he was too much for any one caregiver to physically handle.

Sandra had gone back to her life in New Orleans; Susie was probably starting her sophomore year in high school. I remember I had a job lined up for the ski season at Dercum's Ski Tip Ranch near Arapahoe Basin, Colorado. The job didn't start until the end of October. I don't remember what David was doing or where he was working. I do know he had graduated from University of Northern Iowa and found a placeholder job in Waterloo while he actively searched for something better.

Meanwhile, I watched Mother closely for signs of another nervous breakdown. She seemed depressed and somewhat despondent.

Otherwise, she seemed to be holding her own. Dad, on the other hand, had quit practicing psychiatry and spent most days unshaven and holed up in his den with the door closed, a glass and a bottle of Kentucky rye for company. What he did in there for hours on end neither Mother nor I could figure out. He had now become one of the "unreachables."

One early afternoon, a week before I was to take off for Colorado, I walked into the kitchen to find Mother and Dad wrestling with a loaded pistol. No screaming. Just the guttural struggle of one will against another. Panicked, I wrestled the gun from them and said, "If you kill her, I swear to God, I'll kill you." Afterwards, I ran from the house and hid the gun at Janice's.

A few nights later, Dad came to my room. I had just drifted off, but woke fully to his silhouette framed by the hall light. I couldn't see his face. Perched gingerly on the edge of my bed, his back bent round like the letter C, he held my hand and apologized for the episode with the loaded gun, and for never telling us kids straight-out about Mother's hospitalization all those years ago, even for never paying me much attention. Sandra had always been Dad's favorite of the girls, and Bill his north star. And he was sorry, so sorry, about Bill. Said it was all his fault. That he should never have pushed Bill into pre-med when all he wanted was to be an artist. "Believe me Ginny, I love you. Really. Will you forgive me?"

"I don't know what to believe, Dad." I pulled back my hand. "Besides, it's too late for Bill." I rolled onto my side, away from him, away from his too little, too late apology. He had been so engaged playing savior at work, plucking the lives of strangers from their oceanic abyss, that he had lost sight of those who were drowning right under his own roof.

The next day Janice and I drove to Aspen. I drove like a wild-woman—couldn't put the miles between me and my family fast enough. David wouldn't arrive for another month, but I couldn't wait. I had to escape the craziness at home. Janice and I found a simple, cheap motel with a pool and a convenience store down the street that sold elk jerky, Coors, Fritos and Fudgsicles.

September was nearing its end. Cool nights opened into days cool in the shade, but hot in the sun. Janice and I chose sun and Grizzly Lake, away from road noise, and motel traffic. I nosed the car into a somewhat secluded spot that kept the seats shaded and left the windows down with the radio tuned up. Those afternoons, I nearly forgot about Waterloo, brother Bill, the abortion, my parents. Life was better than good. I could breathe. And the knots that had formed in my gut, the tightness in my chest, the fist jammed in my throat, all but melted in the late summer sun.

One scorching day near the end of September, Janice and I sat in aluminum, webbed lawn chairs, our butts in the lake and our Coors submersed in a nearby pocket of cold runoff. Slouched, with heads back, legs outstretched, we idled, letting the Doors *Light My Fire* wash over us. Liquid, languid stars of light shone behind my closed eyelids. With my body warmed all the way through, I floated the wave of each note, breath rising and falling, serene . . . until the song was interrupted by the announcer's voice asking anyone who knew Ginny Tice to have her immediately call the Aspen Police Station.

David took care of everything. He called Sandra in New Orleans and found me in Aspen and sat with mother while the police trooped through the house and the coroner came and went.

Fortunately, he had been at the house picking up some things I'd asked him to bring me when he heard the gunshot. The bedroom doors had been locked, so David grabbed a painter's ladder and climbed through an open bedroom window. He found the .357 Magnum next to Dad who was half naked, lying between bathroom and bedroom.

Blood and brains spattered the walls and carpet.

Mother had been in the garden pruning roses and said her knees had simply given way when she heard the gunshot, as if it were meant to drop her instead of Dad. David found her, pruning shears still in hand, in a heap on the grass, unable to stand on her own. He helped her up and carried her to the front porch where they waited for the police.

In the wake of Dad's suicide, Sandra quit her job and left her beau in New Orleans to move home and care for Susie and Mother. Susie was fifteen, a sophomore in high school and, while broken-hearted, she was resilient. I cannot say the same for Mother. She slept all hours of the day and night and when awake she was rarely out of her housedress. Weekly hair appointments were missed, as were country club engagements that had been on her calendar for months. Brother Bill, ever foremost on Mother's agenda with daily visits, was forgotten, or not forgotten so much as given over to the care of the nursing home professionals who "obviously know more about his care than I do." She instructed us to tell friends who called that she was "unavailable", then stared for hours at the cold blank screen of the television. Sandra cajoled her into a few spoonfuls of soup on occasion, but it wasn't enough. Mother's clothes began to hang off her like some emaciated mannequin. Within a month, we knew it was time.

One wet and grey October day, Sandra and I got Susie off to school, then bathed and carefully dressed Mother in her favorite navy suit, cream silk blouse, pearls, hose and pumps. We told her we all needed some fresh air. For a woman who had refused to leave the house or talk to anyone but us three girls for nearly a month, she was surprisingly compliant as Sandra and I folded her gently into the back seat of the Lincoln Continental.

Sandra sat in back with Mother and held her thin hand as I aimed the Lincoln south to Cedar Rapids. Sandra chatted with her as though we were on a girl's afternoon out—lunch and a few quick stops to pick up things at Younkers in Cedar Rapids before heading home.

Mother didn't say a word when I pulled into the porte-cochère at Mercy Hospital, or when an orderly stepped through the glass doors pushing a wheelchair, or when the heavy metal door in the locked ward clicked shut behind us, or when she took in the white-on-white of her room, or when the nurse unfastened Mother's pearls and handed them to Sandra. Not a word.

We had no choice.

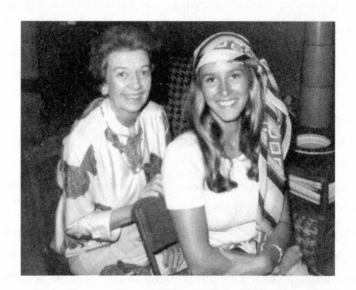

MY BEAUTIFUL, TROUBLED MOTHER, PEARL
TICE, AND ME. SHE STRUGGLED WITH MENTAL
ILLNESS FOR AS LONG AS I CAN REMEMBER.
AFTER DAD'S SUICIDE SHE WAS NEVER THE SAME.
(WATERLOO, IOWA, 1969)

NEW ORLEANS, LOUISIANA

SEPTEMBER 1972

BY 1972, DAVID AND I HAD BEEN MARRIED for a few years and living like gypsies—Iowa, Wisconsin, Indiana, Long Island—each time for some new job opportunity David thought would be "the one." David had fantasies of becoming a millionaire by thirty, while I just wanted to settle down in one spot long enough to establish myself as an artist. I'd been drawing and painting since I was four. In a relatively short time, wherever we landed, I made inroads into the art community, selling a few notecards, prints, and calendars. Then along would come David's next big opportunity to sweep it all away.

I was sick of moving and being dependent. The Podunk towns, the cabin in Green Bay, Wisconsin without running water. The isolation of making art on a Formica table in some windowless, airless apartment, while David navigated his way to successively better jobs for bigger paychecks with men who would shake his hand, wish him luck, and tell him he would be sorely missed when he gave notice.

My luck changed when David landed a position as Sales Manager at the Royal Sonesta Hotel in the French Quarter in my beloved New Orleans. A window opened and I jumped. David and I immersed ourselves in the French Quarter, the nightlife and bar scene. I drew and painted during the days, and began making a name for myself and my art. I was asked to model—runway and print. One contact led to the next. One night in Bruno's Bar a movie producer offered me a role as a body double for Suzy Kendall in the 1972 B movie, *Fear is the Key*. I took it, then a few months later I drove and rolled a stunt car in the James Bond movie, *Live and Let Die*. Movies led to television commercials. One morning when the guy I was to pitch with didn't show up, I called David. With his clean-cut good looks, the producers hired him on the spot.

David and I became the "in" couple in the French Quarter. People pointed us out, bought us drinks. We moved in the stratosphere of the French Quarter, oblivious to the ordinary, and intoxicated with ourselves. Amongst the cadre of people who flowed with us, Sandra and her boyfriend often tagged along. Often the boyfriend was Bob Levi.

Bob did not know the meaning of "no." Instead, he saw "no," as the gauntlet thrown. In crowded, noisy bars it was relatively easy to keep space between myself and Bob, particularly when he was with Sandra. However, he found out where David and I lived and knew David's hours at Royal Sonesta. He began sending roses, pink and deep red. I threw them out. Next arrived gifts, including a silk scarf with horses. I loved it. I wore it everywhere and had David asked, I'd have said I bought it myself. Next came a gold bracelet, which I kept but did not wear. I called and asked how his wife and kids were and told him to stop. He did not.

Instead, Bob approached David about a fifty-fifty partnership in a new hotel in Slidell, Louisiana—Bob would front the cash and David would run it. David, unaware of Bob's mafia connections or advances towards me, thought it was a great opportunity. Bob was getting way out of hand. At my urging, David began looking for other opportunities and found one as Manager of Pine Valley Ranch in Pine, Colorado.

That opportunity, while it did not last, at least got us away from Bob. The problem was, it also took me away from the excitement and connections and life I cherished in New Orleans. The ranch was as lonely as all those Podunk towns and airless apartments had been during our first years of marriage.

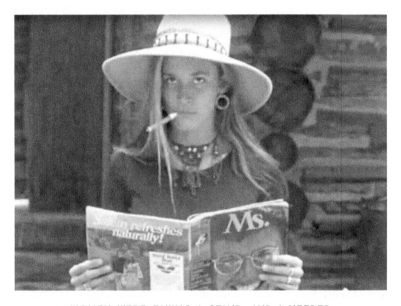

WOMEN WERE TAKING A STAND, AND I NEEDED TO AS WELL. MY MARRIAGE TO DAVID NEEDED PROTECTION. TO GET AWAY FROM BOB LEVI AND HIS SEDUCTIVE, FAST-PACED MAFIA LIFE, I COAXED MY HUSBAND TO SEEK WORK ELSEWHERE. PERHAPS WE COULD REINVENT OURSELVES, BUT SOON I GREW RESTLESS.
(PINE, COLORADO, 1973)

David's next move, now that he was enamored with ranch life, took us to the second-largest dude ranch in the state, Paradise Ranch, which lay at the foot of Pike's Peak near Colorado Springs. Within six months, the owners were found to be embezzling, so we moved on. This time to Fort Worth, Texas for a job with Dell Webb Land Development, selling lots in Dell's newest project in ~~Grand Lake,~~ Colorado. Granby, CO

By this time, I was not only lonely, but depressed and disenchanted with our lifestyle and the marriage. Don't get me wrong, I loved David. He had been there for every family crisis in 1969 and never once ducked out on me. Always he was by my side, quiet, steady, helping in any way he could. But the gypsy life and my isolation were getting old. New Orleans had been the perfect mix for us. David and I had each pursued our passions. I had carved out my own niche and was rapidly building a career in fashion and art. We had escaped Bob, but following in David's wake left me lonely and dependent.

Following Mother's second nervous breakdown, she had been anxious to get out from under the pall of our Waterloo home. New Orleans was the obvious choice—near Sandra, who was the only one of us girls who was settled—and Mother had always loved New Orleans. Early in my parents' marriage, until I was four-and-a-half years old, Dad had taught neurology at Tulane University. Mother, an Iowa native, had embraced the South wholeheartedly. With three children, she loved having help—a cook, nanny, and gardener were affordable on a professor's salary in the late 40s early 50s. After so many years away, it thrilled her to be returning.

We found Mother the perfect home on Lake Vista, one designed by a student of Frank Lloyd Wright. On the lake side of the house, brick window boxes spilled over with begonia blossoms and doors opened onto a brick patio with a water feature and built-in barbeque. Rose bushes edged the sunny side of the patio. A magnificent Live Oak held bird feeders in which the squirrels hung upside down to feed. Mother loved it. Once she was firmly ensconced in New Orleans with Sandra nearby, I didn't think too much about her. I had never quite forgiven her for leaving us when I was nine to go on her "vacation." Even once I knew the truth and came to a better understanding of mental illness, it still rankled that any mother could just walk away from her kids for nine months. So, it came as a surprise in November of 1972, when I had a foreboding dream that something had happened to her.

A quick call to Sandra confirmed that overnight Mother had had a heart attack. Sandra was on her way to the hospital, while Mother awaited surgery for a pacemaker. I caught the first flight to New Orleans and she was on the operating table by the time my plane touched down. It seemed I spent more time sitting vigil in hospitals than living my life. When I began to add it up, Mother's litany of illness was astounding—the nervous breakdowns in 1958 and 1969 were just the culminations of other more nebulous conditions—a thyroid problem (too low) that never seemed to improve, bouts with depression, a fidgety anxiety that drove the help crazy. Some housekeepers stuck it out for a year or more. Most gave notice within six months. Gardeners, being men and outdoors, tended to last longer.

As family and daughters, Sandra, Susie and I couldn't quit. I wasn't sure how Sandra and Susie felt, but I wanted to. This heart attack was so typically Mother. Every time I managed to create some distance between us, some new illness would arise to reel me back to her side.

A few days later, while sitting vigil with Mother in the hospital, I received a note from Bob Levi. He was waiting for me in the bar across the street.

I took the elevator down and walked across the rain-slick street to meet him. Bob had my usual on the table—a gin and tonic with the tonic chilling in an ice bucket at his side. He stood as I approached, watched me walk across the room as if I were the only woman in it and deftly seated me. I hadn't remembered him as quite this handsome, although it had only been a little over a year since I'd seen him. He wore a dark blue suit, a light blue starched button-down shirt, burgundy tie expertly knotted, knife creases on the trousers, and a matching hankie in the blazer pocket. To spite the late afternoon, he didn't have any five-o'clock shadow and every wavy black hair on his head was in place. To sum Bob up in a word: crisp. He didn't waste time on small talk. He told me he had always loved me. Wanted to be with me, not Sandra, not his wife, not anyone else.

I was swaying like the tallest of poplars in the fall wind. I had married David for surety and security. David offered emotional stability that, no matter how many times we moved, or whatever happened in my crazy family, he was always there. David was predictable, dependable in a way that I sensed a man like Bob never would be. Bob had always felt dangerous and because he felt dangerous, I had always gone in the other direction. This time something felt different, not with Bob, but with me, so when Bob swore he would divorce his wife and stop seeing Sandra, I almost believed him. Because I wanted to.

I sipped the gin and tonic as Bob slipped a small white jewelers' box from his suit pocket. With an index finger, he slid it across the table. Inside lay, not the ring I dreaded, but a gold house key. I glanced up from the key, impressed by his moxie, yet floored. "I'm not living with you, Bob."

"Fine. For now." Bob threw back the rest of his whiskey. "You're horsey, right? Let's take a ride out to the farm in Folsom and I'll show you around."

NEW ORLEANS, LOUISIANA

1975

LAST TIME UP'S PHOTO FINISH IN HER FIRST race had proven a woman could train a racehorse and I was just getting started. The hitch: Bob owned her. Given the contentious nature of our relationship over the last four-and-a-half years, now that he had something I loved, I wouldn't have put it past him to use the filly as leverage to keep me in the relationship.

After Bob divorced his wife, I divorced David and moved in with Bob on the farm in Folsom. I still loved David, but couldn't go back to Texas. I yearned for the kind of tangible stability Bob could provide—a beautifully appointed and staffed home, thoroughbred racehorses right outside the door, fine dining and dinner parties. The ease of life Bob could provide with his wealth and power outweighed stringing along behind David from one job to the next until he supposedly hit it big. And the sex—Bob had a rare condition that kept him going well beyond the limits of other men—both a blessing and a curse. A lure almost as powerful as the horses. I may have left David for Bob, but I stayed for the land and the horses, especially the horses, not for Bob.

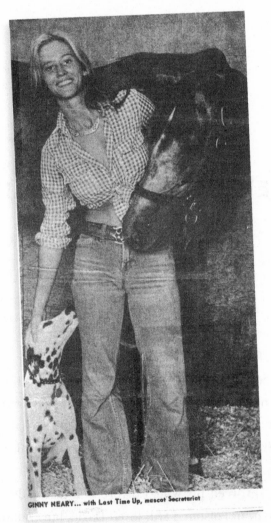

GINNY NEARY... with Last Time Up, mascot Secretariat

I WAS THE FIRST WOMAN LICENSED IN LOUISIANA TO TRAIN THOROUGHBRED RACE HORSES. IN 1975, A NEWSPAPER PHOTOGRAPHER TOOK THIS PHOTO OF ME SANDWICHED BETWEEN MY DALMATION, SECRETARIAT, AND THOROUGHBRED RACE HORSE, LAST TIME UP. THE PHOTO WAS TAKEN AT JIMMIE ERWIN'S TRAINING CENTER IN FOLSOM, LOUISIANA. A PROUD MOMENT FOR ME.

Over our time together, I left Bob roughly every six months, fleeing to David or to Mother's place on Lake Vista, or in a pinch moving into a trailer on the farm. I couldn't seem to stand up to Bob. He was dismissive, patronizing. Yet I wouldn't let him keep me down either. Often, while in Folsom I fled to my dear surrogate family, the Pittmans. Southern Baptists though they were, they still loved me and overlooked the fact I lived with the likes of Bob—no small thing. It became a daily stop to have lunch at Ma Pittmans. Their daughter, Jane, the local high school gym teacher, became a good friend.

Often, before I went to Ma Pittman's, I would stop at the Tautog thoroughbred farm owned by my dear friend Geraldine Fitzsimmons. Geraldine was also my first important collector of art. She was a sophisticated, well-to-do woman from New York City, with horses in her background—primarily jumpers. I was honored that she liked my art. She was not a fan of Bob Levi. We would talk of all things on her back porch, sipping, usually, iced tea. She had four young boys, one a newborn. These people were also part of my family, very important for my stability. It is interesting that we still talk by Skype— Geraldine in Montana, having left after Hurricane Katrina, and me in Patagonia—every week.

But even the stable resource of their home and friendship couldn't override the stress of the constant game of push-me-pull-you I had with Bob and Last Time Up. This was not a game I wanted to play. The language Bob truly understood was money, so I asked him to name his price. He did: three grand.

Every penny I had. What the hell else was I going to do with three grand? Three grand wouldn't support me if I left him or buy me a piece of land or any other appreciable investment. As fickle as fate tied to a horse can be, Last Time Up was my best bet.

The filly's second race was at Jefferson Downs in Kenner, Louisiana, a suburb of New Orleans. Competition was stiffer and it was a $5000 claiming race. A "claim" meant that anyone who had an interest in a horse *plus* the cash could file a claim in the race secretary's office prior to the race. Whatever the outcome, win or lose, place or show, dead or alive, the horse was theirs. Safe bet, I thought. No one would claim a horse yet to win a race.

Bob and I each bet $100 across the board and $10 on jockey and gateman for a total payout of $68 mutual. In English—every two-dollar bet recouped $68. A lot of dough.

This was a night race, with bright lights and a track with limited vision—nothing Last Time Up was used to. My hands shook as I saddled her and gave my jockey, Mike Keller, a leg up. Mike made his own adjustments and loaded smoothly into the gate. The buzzer sounded

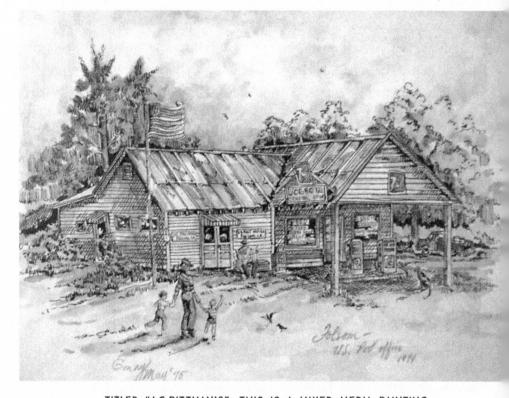

TITLED "J.C.PITTMAN'S", THIS IS A MIXED MEDIA PAINTING BY ME (PEN & INK WATERCOLOR) DEPICTING GERALDINE FITZSIMMONS WITH TWO OF HER BOYS, GOING TO J.C. PITTMAN'S GENERAL STORE AND GAS STATION/POST OFFICE IN FOLSOM, LOUISIANA, 1974.

and the latch sprung. They were off. Last Time Up leapt to the lead and never glanced back. I screamed, "Go, go, go," the entire race and prayed no one had placed a claim on her.

At the window, the cashier handed me more hundred-dollar bills than I had ever seen. I didn't have enough pockets, purse, anything to contain them. Panicked by the thought I'd be mugged, I stuffed money down my jodhpurs and bra while Bob laughed, stuffing his own pockets fat to overflowing.

A quick check-in at the secretary's office revealed Last Time Up had not been claimed. I had a load of money and still owned my filly. Perfect.

The next day, Mr. Cleat and I combed over the *Condition Book* to find the next race and singled out another one at Jefferson Downs. Three-quarters of a mile. The competition was stiff and the purses fatter. I gambled that no one would put in a $7500 claim on Last Time Up, but was nervous after her last stellar performance.

After some time off, I began three weeks of conditioning to build her back up to perfect form. With race day looming, Last Time Up put in a breakneck workout and Mr. Cleat and I agreed she was at her peak. I arrived at the track two hours early for another night race. At least now the lights would be familiar, but there were so many other variables—the filly's nerves fueled by other horses' whinnying and stamping, the track noise, the loudspeaker, loose programs fluttering across the racetrack and a thousand other unknowns over which I had no control.

"Horses to the paddock," blasted through the PA system.

Last Time Up was dressed to thrill in her white racing bridle and she knew it as she pranced in place. Mike Keller was standing by in his silks, all smiles with racing saddle in hand. I walked the filly around the paddock a few times, then led her into the stall to saddle her. "Mike this is your second time on her. You know what she can do."

Mike hadn't lost that grin. He nodded and said, "You bet."

"Riders up."

I gave Mike a leg up and stepped back. Our fate was in his hands now. Win or lose, this horse was ready. Last Time Up loaded well into the gate while others balked or refused. From the grandstand, my filly looked small and miles away. I bet big. Laid down $100 across the board as did Bob. I placed bets for Mike at $10 across the board and $10 on the gateman so he wouldn't be inclined to hold her tail, thereby curbing her break. As Evangeline Downs proved, races can be won or lost depending on how a horse breaks from the gate.

At the bell, Last Time Up flew to the lead. My heart felt like it was going to rupture as I watched a gelding gain and stick with her, nose to her tail. Another filly began inching up almost even with her, then Mike asked for that final burst of speed and Last Time Up joyously complied, pulling ahead for the win. I glanced at the mutual board. She had put in a blistering time.

Claimed, or not? I was afraid to check.

The winner's circle was a blur. Mike and his wife were there, Bob, Mr. Cleat, the presenter, ribbon, photos, and the smiles and smiles before the tears at learning Last Time Up had indeed been claimed. Of course, I got the $7500 in claim money and the winnings were huge, but I couldn't afford to buy her back. All the way home I fought nausea at the finality of this loss. In the days following, a wrenching tightness gripped my chest each time I passed her empty stall. I hadn't just lost a horse, I'd lost a friend.

My only solace was the winnings gave me enough financial independence that I could leave Bob and his pastel Cadillac and shady business deals and his mafia buddies who came and went under a thin veil of the pretense of doing business. But was it ever complicated. As much as I hated Bob's under the table deals and acquaintances, I did love him. Just as I was ready to bolt, with one foot out the door, another filly, Cajun Cousin, needed my attention ... plus the mare, Giggles, was due to foal in January. Reasons to stick around a bit longer.

I stayed with Bob by managing to keep busy enough that we really didn't spend too much alone time together. Together, we entertained his mob friends, associates and their girlfriends, never the wives. The trade-off was that by staying in one place for over four years, I had built not only a reputation as a serious and skilled trainer, but as a fine equestrian artist.

As with most successes, I came by this one through the backdoor. It started with a gig as Art Director for *Louisiana Horse Magazine*. It took my small staff and I hours a week to roll out, copy, and literally cut and paste the magazine together. In my calls to sell ad space, I met some of the movers and shakers in Louisiana's horse scene. Inspired by their stories, I began to paint portraits of their horses. That garnered me a monthly full-color, full-page spread for my equestrian art and I began to make a name for myself, first in the South, then later nationwide through *The Horseman's Journal*.

Bob must have sensed my ambivalence regarding our relationship, because with his winnings from Last Time Up's race, he bought me a mink jacket. It wasn't my style, but it was classy and in good taste, with a suede sash and my name embroidered on the jacket's satin lining.

Six weeks later, right before Christmas, Bob took Mother and me to dinner in the French Quarter, then on to the Roosevelt Hotel's Sazerac Bar to see Frankie Laine. While waiting for the show to start, he presented Mother and me with our Christmas gifts. For Mother, a gold bracelet set with sapphires. She giggled and her cheeks flushed. For me, a ring with a two-carat emerald encircled in diamonds. My god! He thought he could buy me? Yet he made Mother so happy with his gifts, which were always expensive and thoughtful. And it did feel good to still be pursued after nearly four years of our relationship running hot and cold. He made it easy to forget the difference between security and love.

The day after New Year's, Giggles foaled. It was early morning; cold. The mare was heaving, pushing, the foal stuck. By the time the vet arrived, the little filly was up, but refusing to nurse. I tried to help her latch on to the teat, but she showed no interest, instead she staggered across the stall on her stick legs and bumped into the wall as if she didn't see it. After several hours of observation, the vet, worried about brain damage, advised Bob to put the foal down.

Giggles wasn't a first-time mother. She poked and prodded her foal, nickered and nudged, becoming upset at her foal's lack of instinct to latch on. I was crying and running my hands over the foal while Bob weighed the vet's advice. This was a valuable foal. Other than not nursing, she had good confirmation—straight legs, promising haunches, a well-proportioned neck and head. The filly staggered. Bob lifted his cap, ran a hand through his wavy black hair, sighed and pulled the cap down hard. He called for Melvin, a gimpy but dependable ranch hand, and said, "Dig a hole."

I begged Bob to give me a day, just one, to see if I could get the foal to nurse. Bob looked from me to the vet. The vet said, "I can't make the decision for you, Bob. It's your money."

"One day, Ginny."

Alone with the mare and foal, I did the only thing I could think of—I milked the mare, who accommodated my cold shaking hands. She seemed to know I was trying to help. By the time I had the colostrum, or first milk, the filly had folded to the ground. I sat in the straw and lifted her head to my lap, keeping her neck long while nudging a turkey baster with the colostrum into the corner of her mouth. She gagged. I knew I could drown her, but without the milk, she'd be dead anyway, so I kept at it until her eyes closed in sleep. With her head in my lap, I leaned back against the barn wall and dozed off.

An hour later the foal woke and struggled to stand. With her mother's nickering and nosing and my pulling and bracing, she eventually stood and found her own balance, but was still unable to nurse. I milked Giggles and fed the foal throughout the day and late into the night. Mother, baby and I were all exhausted. I laid down with them in the stall and we slept.

In the morning, Bob and the vet were amazed to find the foal still alive. Bob gave me another day, then another. By the third day he said, "Ginny, you've earned her. I'll bring home the papers tomorrow and if she's still alive, she's yours."

NEW ORLEANS, LOUISIANA

SEPTEMBER 1976

DESPITE BOB AND HIS MOB BULLSHIT and our push-me-pull-you relationship, I felt life was finally going my way. I was making it as an equine artist, as a racehorse trainer in a man's world, and, due to Last Time Up's wins, I had my own money in the bank so I didn't have to beg it from Bob like some schoolgirl asking for allowance.

The magic spell broke when Mother was hospitalized with intestinal cancer. Surgery that removed a foot-and-a-half of intestine meant she was in the hospital for a good month. During that time, I commuted thirty-minutes each way from Folsom across Lake Pontchartrain to the hospital in New Orleans. Twenty-seven miles on the causeway over all that water is monotonous, hypnotic. One day, on my way back to the farm, my mind spun—thinking of Mother's anxiety, the absence of a foot-and-a-half of her intestine, colostomy bag, yes or no, horses under saddle, Bob's latest gift—a motorcycle for God's sake—and before I knew it, my chin snapped up from my chest. I jerked the steering wheel hard, just missing the guardrail and a swim in Lake Pontchartrain.

A week later, I was running late to the barn to meetup with Mr. Cleat and exercise my filly. I hurriedly loaded my Dalmatian pup, Secretariat, into the back of the pickup along with some tack and took off. When I arrived, no dog. Damn it. I retraced my route, but didn't see him. Deciding the motorcycle would make a better search vehicle for the deep woods, I floored it for home, grabbed the bike, then headed back down the road. After twenty minutes of searching and calling, I glimpsed a flash of white off to the side in a deep ditch, and there lay Secretariat, who lifted his head, but was otherwise paralyzed. I had run over my own dog and broken his pelvis. *Good lord*, I thought, *how could that have happened?*

Another ten days went by. Secretariat was in his cast and now rode shotgun on the front seat in the mornings as I headed to the barn. I loved training thoroughbred racehorses—winning the horse's respect, teaching the horse to give what's asked, then asking a little more, the sensing when to push or when to pull back and give a skill just a little more time, the thrill of the speed on the morning exercise runs, the sweat and muscle. No effort was too much, so when I was asked to exercise a gelding I didn't know, I agreed.

There was something about that horse I didn't like. I couldn't quite put my finger on what it was and started to reconsider. But there was Mr. Cleat, horse bridled, reins in hand, waiting. I threw my saddle on and Mr. Cleat gave me a leg up. "Okay, Sweet Ginny Lee, once around to warm up, then give him a solid workout. Fast as he can for a quarter mile."

The warmup went all right, but when I let him open up to run, he was reluctant. I coaxed him on and he almost pulled it together for a few strides before he began to crumble under me, collapsing through the inside rail. I fell, one foot caught in the stirrup. The leathers didn't release and as he thrashed, his hooves just missed my chest and grazed my helmet. The gelding crashed back through the inside rail, taking the homestretch at a full gallop with me dangling from the stirrup or at least a hundred yards. When the stirrup finally released, I clamored up, brushing dirt from eyes, nose, mouth. "I'm fine," I told Mr. Cleat. But the look on his face told me I shouldn't be.

The next day was Friday. I was bruised and stiff, but I'd have the weekend to recover. I was twenty-seven, no problem. Except my quiet weekend was usurped by Bob's last-minute plans for a weekend-long house party with some of his mafia friends from New Orleans. Around the pool late on Saturday afternoon, Bob hounded me to show off my new motorcycle to his two buddies who'd ridden in on their bikes. When I rolled up on my bike, the guys were revving theirs, showing off and popping wheelies. Over the roar of their engines, I couldn't hear how much I'd revved my own bike and my foot jerked, popping the clutch. Fast decision. Two ways to fall: backwards into the metal-framed lawn chairs on the pavement, or forward into the pool.

As I sank, I remembered the sound of the engine as it slowly sputtered out and the dull resonance still reverberating in my ears as they filled with water. I let go when I touched bottom and pushed to the surface. "Are you mad, Bob?"

Bob stood with his mouth open, running a hand through his hair until a buddy filled it with a drink. "Jesus, Ginny. Just. Jesus."

Our house party rolled on through the evening with many jovial and good-natured ribs about my "stunt ride." Lots of slaps on the back for Bob for landing such a rebel. Truth is, it was an accident and, being an accident, it scared the hell out of me. I had no idea how my foot involuntarily jerked and popped the clutch, but I was never going to admit that. Better to let these guys worship the legacy of my 007 stunt drive and view this accident as performance.

Sunday's squirrel hunt was the event everyone had come for. Can't do that in the city. Despite their hangovers, the guys were out early on foot, tramping through the brush, dogs scenting, howling when they'd treed a squirrel. Men yelling. A shot. Another. I was foot-dragging tired. The only reason I went out was that I had a reputation to live up to. If I had stayed behind with the women, these guys would have assumed the little woman couldn't handle a gun. False. Dad had taught me well. The crew was at least a quarter mile ahead, so I found a tree-shaded spot and sat cross-legged on the ground, resting the shotgun across my lap. After half an hour or so, I figured I'd better rejoin the group before anyone was the wiser. Oddly, my legs had fallen asleep. No big deal. Just shake them out and wait a few minutes for the pins and needles to subside. Except, they didn't. By lunch, I couldn't feel a thing in my left leg—hip to foot—and not much in my right.

Monday morning, I lay in bed, ticking off the list of barn chores: horses to exercise, the cutting and pasting to be done at the magazine, the drive to New Orleans to visit Mother in the hospital. The day was already too short. Then Bob's hand cupped my breast. "No. Not enough time," I said. But this was Bob and, as always, he persisted until I gave in. But this was different. When I went to wrap my left arm around his back, I couldn't lift it. In fact, I couldn't feel him inside me. Couldn't feel anything on the entire left side of my body—ear, shoulder, breast, hip, knee, toes. Nothing.

Bob drove me to Touro Infirmary. I was poked and prodded and run through test after test for over a month before the doctors finally determined that it could be either a brain tumor or Multiple Sclerosis. Those were the days before MRIs (Magnetic Resonance Imaging). A brain tumor could not be confirmed without cutting into the brain, while Multiple Sclerosis, or MS, was one of those diseases that couldn't be diagnosed. Instead, it was a process of elimination, testing for and ruling out known diseases until doctors were left with a handful that most closely matched the patient's symptoms. With nothing to lose, my doctor put me on an intravenous drip of ACTH, a form of Prednisone and a powerful anti-inflammatory. Thankfully, I responded, but the doctor was still reluctant to confirm a diagnosis of MS.

Initially, Bob was by my side in the hospital, even slept there, but after the first month, he begged off, citing work and two ex-wives and their children to support. My friend Jane later told me that within days of my hospitalization, Bob had called her to the house. The den was dark, shuttered against the late afternoon sun. Bob sat with *The Encyclopedia Britannica* open on the coffee table in front of him, head in his hands. The page heading: Multiple Sclerosis. Through tears, Bob said he was going to marry me. Take care of me no matter what.

The second month, my sister Susie picked up the slack at the hospital. Living at my place, she drove into town daily to keep me company. I was lucky the paralysis had only affected my left side, allowing me to continue drawing and painting . . . until the morning I woke to my right side numb. Unable to open and close my right hand, I ranted and railed. By the end of the day I was completely paralyzed. I could no longer brush my hair or teeth or hold a paint brush or coffee cup.

I unloaded on anyone who would listen, especially my doctor. Was this permanent? I was an artist for God's sake. I didn't have time for this. I mean, I could possibly give up riding or even walking, but drawing and painting? Impossible. This was twenty-first century medicine, couldn't they do something? Science sent people to the moon. Defied gravity. There had to be something someone could do, some new discovery, or a wonder drug awaiting FDA approval. But day in, day out, my doctor's answer was the same: "We'll just have to wait and see."

Multiple Sclerosis is mysterious, unpredictable. MS occurs when myelin, a protective fatty coating around nerves in the brain and spinal cord, is destroyed. This destruction interrupts and distorts nerve impulses to the brain. This disease is called Multiple because many areas of the brain and spinal cord are affected and Sclerosis because of the sclerosed, or scar, tissue that forms at damaged sites.

Some people have one minor bout and regain function. Others go into remission then relapse, cycling through relapse-remission over the course of years. Still others remain permanently paralyzed. Given the severity of my attack, doctors thought permanent paralyzation was likely. If I was lucky enough to regain function, I was warned it could take a year or more. Even so, my doctor and those with whom he conferred, would not commit to a firm diagnosis.

All the news about MS was bad. The doctors offered little in the way of constructive solutions for recovery. They knew nothing about whether physical therapy would help. The best they had to offer was, "it couldn't hurt." No advice on nutrition. Nothing. Their advice on lifestyle—slow down. I laughed. I was twenty-seven. I had no intention of slowing down or giving in to this disease.

One evening, my childhood friend, Janice, called and told me the only good news I ever heard about MS. An acquaintance of hers with MS said every Christmas the stress of the holidays incited a relapse and she'd wind up in a wheelchair, but by the end of February or March, she'd go into complete remission and be up and walking, even skiing again. I decided if that woman could do it, so could I.

I was in Touro Infirmary for three months, during which time Susie kept vigil. Sandra, Bob and a host of friends were in and out. A friend of Susie's flew down from Iowa, a native Iowan with an easy way, quick smile, and milky-smooth complexion. She was with us at the hospital one afternoon when Bob dropped by. Four of us occupied the room, however the energy in it coalesced around Bob and Susie's friend. I knew the look on his face too well. I knew that sparkle in the eye, the half-smile, lips oozing smooth Southern charm. Shit. I hoped I was wrong.

The day the roses started arriving, I knew. Susie's teary arrival a bit later that morning confirmed my hunch. A few days later, Bob showed up and pushed in through the riot of color and fragrance and thorns, begging my forgiveness. On his knees, next to my hospital bed, he kissed the back of my paralyzed right hand, then slipped a Tiffany engraved silver I.D. bracelet around my wrist. The engraving read, "Love You."

"Get out, Bob."

"Ginny, please." Fat tears welled at the rims of his eyes, then flooded his cheeks. "I couldn't help myself. I need . . . and you just . . . what I mean is . . . well, you're . . ."

"Paralyzed. The word is paralyzed, Bob." I heard the tone of my words, flat, as if observing the scene unfolding from a distance, perhaps from the third-row center aisle in a dark theatre. I wanted the woman on the screen to tell this man to piss off. Rise up against the odds and out of that hospital bed. Walk out the damn door. Leave him on his knees at her bedside with his crocodile tears.

But the lights came up and the rage and humiliation settled heavy into my useless body. So much to say, but I couldn't say a word and lowered my eyelids.

"Come back to the ranch, to Folsom. The horses need you. I need you."

Easier with my eyes closed. "I need you," resonated in the hollow where love wanted to be. Or was. I wasn't sure. I missed the horses and Mr. Cleat and the way this man's smell sent adrenaline washing through my system, giving me the feeling that anything, anything at all, was possible. That life was rich and silken gold as honey and just waiting for me to step up and take my place.

"I'll think on it." My eyes were still mercifully shuttered against Bob; my senses avoiding the hospital room smelling faintly of disinfectant and boldly of roses in all states of bloom and decay.

The day I was finally sprung from the hospital, I went home to Mother's on Lake Vista. I was still bedridden and needed a walker or wheelchair, but was definitely regaining some mobility. Mother had just had her second surgery for intestinal cancer. No one would have guessed. She cared for me, as if her own pain and suffering didn't exist, as if I were the only thing in her world that mattered. She was tender in a way my body remembered. Her hands stayed firm but loving as they held, supported, lifted, lowered, pushed, pulled, brushed, bathed, and fed me. Her voice remained soft, soothing, never irritated or hurried. We had reverted to a simpler time where the roles of mother and daughter were as clear as they had been when I was an infant and then a small child with croup, gasping for air, a time when I had looked to her to provide comfort for us both.

Parked in the sun on Mother's patio, I'd wheel over to a sturdy post and pulled myself up, trying to walk by bracing my hands on walls and chairs. I sweated and swore those first days, but after a few weeks began to feel the strength in my arms and legs build. I knew I was going to be fine, better than fine. I kept visualizing the barn at Folsom, Mr. Cleat, the three horses in training, my drawing and painting.

Eight months after that first attack, I returned to the barn at Folsom to train. I no longer galloped the horses, but being with them daily hastened my recovery. I found strength without willing it. Thinking about them, focusing on their training plans, races, and breeding rather than myself, gave me a renewed sense of purpose and determination. I began to make gains at a rate that surprised

VIRGINIA NEARY CARRITHERS

the doctors and fed my fire to heal. After a year and a half, I was in remission, ninety percent healed and riding again.

NEW ORLEANS, LOUISIANA

MARCH 1978

IN THE MEANTIME, WITH THE BARN CAME BOB. And with Bob came the persistent pressure to secure a firm diagnosis. He wanted more than anything to know for sure what *we* were dealing with. That bothered me, how he kept using the word *we*. I was the one dealing, not him. David was the one willing to listen as I talked about my daily struggles with this disease. Bob's lack of ease with my illness puzzled me. Despite the fact that he continued to profess his love through extravagant gifts, he couldn't tolerate any mention of MS.

One evening, I turned a corner in the barn, headed toward my truck and home to Mother's in Lake Vista. I nearly bumped into Bob. He stopped, blocking my way, and smiled. Out of the pocket of his leather jacket came a two-carat diamond ring. "I mean to take care of you," he said. Dropping the ring in my shirt pocket, he pivoted on his boot heel and walked away.

Through his connections, Bob found the preeminent neurosurgery center in the country at Baylor University in Houston, Texas. I went. At Baylor, after a week of testing, Dr. Stanley Appel thought I had all the signs of MS and gave me my first official diagnosis, although he warned that so little was understood of the disease that he might be wrong. But MS was likely; highly likely.

With a ring on my finger, I moved back to Folsom and in with Bob. His promise to take care of me, made during those early days of my hospitalization and sworn to my friend Jane, had surprisingly stuck. When I told David, whom I still loved, he married his girlfriend, Sheryl.

Living back at the farm, I wasted no time. If I wasn't with my horses, I was with my art, or entertaining friends and associates with Bob. I felt healthy, vibrant, and alive in a way I'd never experienced. Yes, I was a bit weaker and no, I no longer galloped my own horses, but my horses—Cajun Cousin and Ginny's Little Eva—raced and won. Won big. And requests for my portrait commissions increased.

Weeks turned into months. A film crew did an award-winning documentary on me about living with MS as horsewoman and artist. Editors at the *Times Picayune* and *McCall's* both ran feature articles. Someone at the National Multiple Sclerosis Society noticed all the press and called, asking if I'd be interested in working with them to raise awareness and money for research and patient treatment. The commitment and time involved would be huge. I put them off, waiting for Bob to set a wedding date. I didn't want anything to interfere with our wedding. In the end, I needn't have worried. He never did.

NEW ORLEANS, LOUISIANA

AUGUST 1979

BOTH MEN LOST. A HORSE LOST. No, two horses. In the spring of 1979 Cajun Cousin had been claimed for $7500. As heartbroken as I was to lose her, the timing was good. I needed the money. Multiple Sclerosis is an expensive disease—doctors, Prednisone, physical therapy. That's just for starters. From onset through recovery from my first MS attack, Bob had footed all my medical bills. Now that we were split, the burden fell to me. Me, with no real job, or medical insurance. Me, a quarter-time horse trainer and full-time artist, working when my health allowed. Me, with no dependable income.

The second horse I lost was Ginny's Little Eva. I'd asked Bob several times over the past few years for her papers. Each time it "slipped his mind." In the end, he never signed her over to me. Instead, after saving the life of that foal and training her for more than two years, I watched Bob give her to his new girlfriend. He had helped the woman get her training license, but that didn't make her a trainer. I kept an eye on the filly's races and as far as I know, she never won another. Ginny's Little Eva would not run for my replacement.

In August, I came down with a nasty cold and didn't think much of it until one morning I woke with my feet feeling like quarter-inch cardboard. By early afternoon half-inch cardboard. By evening the sensation had spread up my legs. Another paralysis. I called Dr. Appel in Houston who ordered Prednisone and bedrest. Magic. This time my paralysis wasn't as extensive. It only sidelined me for a month.

Even though I'd made a near full recovery after my first attack, it was becoming clear that my MS was latent and lurking, waiting for the crack in the barn door, the weak hinge on which to pivot and strike. I noticed certain similarities between the two attacks. The first time—Mother was in the hospital; I'd spent long hours at the barn and magazine; there'd been demand for portraits; and then there was my see-saw relationship with Bob. I was doing it all, and doing it all fairly well, but there was a price and it had to be paid somewhere.

This time around I had the loss of both loves, one of the heart and of security, and the other of losing Ginny's Little Eva. So much loss to pile onto the ever-increasing demands on my time and talent. What I had was a deep longing to love and be loved and, through my brother's accident and paralysis and Dad's suicide, a wholehearted compassion for suffering. What I did not have and couldn't see, was that life demanded balance. I had none. From the time my mother was hospitalized when I was nine, I could look back and see that mine was a life of extremes. Always, I was scrambling to close the barn door against the onslaught I thought might be on the other side. As a child, I retreated into nature: drawing, painting and horses. As a young woman, I was still using the tools of a child to manage myself in the world. While I was by any measure successful in the worlds of horse racing, breeding and art, I was failing myself at some deeper level that I'd yet to understand.

EL HEUCÚ, NORTHERN PATAGONIA, ARGENTINA

MARCH 7, 2017

I AM TIRED NOW. ESPECIALLY AFTER I EAT. It seems all the energy my body can muster is required for digestion. This is what life has come down to. Digesting what I have put into it.

Today is my sixty-eighth birthday. You'd think I'd have started with that. To see the big pink candles—a six and an eight—perched next to each other on the top of a four-layer cake, a cake loving crafted by two of my dear caretakers, Rosa and Monica, is a surprise. I never thought I'd live to be this old. After MRIs became available in 1986, I had my first brain scan. The results confirmed, without a doubt, a diagnosis of MS. It was devastating to see multiple lesions on my brain. I had always hoped there'd be some other explanation for my paralysis, something with a cure. Living for ten years without a firm diagnosis had given me hope. Once I knew for certain I had MS, I felt that golden thread of hope slip through my fingers.

A therapist to whom I was referred to in order to deal with my angst, fixed me with a steady gaze and said, "You need to slow down, stop traveling. Set some roots down or you'll be dead at fifty-two." I will never forget the matter-of-fact way he made this pronouncement as I struggled to come to grips with a condition I'd be living with for the rest of my life. I rejected that pronouncement. I ingested that pronouncement. I set out to prove him wrong, but just in case fifty-two was the finish line, I hedged my bets. I resolved to live as if I were one of my racehorses in training. To ask what I could of myself all the time and on the good days, squeeze out just a little more. Giving up is never an option. Although now that I'm confined to my bed and wheelchair, I sometimes think about it.

When my daughter, Sky, and her son, Leo, came to visit recently, we had a talk. At twenty-eight-years-old, Sky is running Ranquilco's cattle operation—100,000 acres—with her partner Chano and two-year-old Leo on her breast, hip and horse. I have no income. She supports me and this chacra in El Heucú, which is no small expense with twenty-four-seven care. I want to contribute but cannot. I can no longer paint. I can no longer ride. My last time up was in 2014 and it took three people to hoist me up and off my grey Arabian. I can feed myself and brush my own teeth and hair. That's the extent of self-sufficiency regarding personal care. I can read very little, as a symptom of MS, retrobulbar neuritis, has affected my eyesight, especially my right eye. The condition is painful and exacerbated by light and especially by any kind of screen time. During flares, I wear an eyepatch and wrap-around dark glasses and try not to think about the pain or wonder whether this time my vision loss will be permanent. So far, each loss over the years has been temporary. My vision has returned, but each time a bit dimmer than the last.

During Sky's visit, I told her I'd be willing to try the nursing home in San Martin de los Andes. San Martin has its pluses. My favorite café is across from the nursing home and just down from the tree-shaded main square, planted in vibrant colors in all seasons. Friends live in San Martin. I would see more of them. I could volunteer in the hospital down the road, coaching art therapy as I once used to when I wintered there. I would need a motorized wheelchair to get around and probably an assistant, just in case. Keeping me in San Martin could possibly cost as much as keeping me here in El Heucú, but with fewer headaches for Sky and no staff to run. My beautiful daughter looked me in the eye and said, "What do *you* want?"

I want to winter in San Martin or Cordoba as I used to. I want to dance. I want to draw and paint and ride the two-and-a-half hours across the cordillera and into Estancia Ranquilco on my grey stallion and live in my rightful place in my home at the corner on the Rio Trocoman. I want to live life on my own terms.

I do not like El Heucú. It is a tiny mountain town in the foothills of the Andes in Northern Patagonia, close to Chile. The people are kind, but simple and lightly educated. No one here speaks any English. The only reason for El Heucú's existence is as a weigh station for the five large estancias and as a spot where many smaller chacras can buy and sell cattle and goats. There are no restaurants or cafes, no cultural life, no art. The streets are dust and businesses still close for siesta every afternoon.

But clearly, what I want and what I need are two different animals—perhaps stallion and elephant. What I have available is consciousness, my daughter, my grandson, my caregivers and this twenty-acre chacra in El Heucú. I have the Lombardi poplars who stand sentry outside my bedroom window, so even on the gloomiest winter days I can watch them dance. I have roses and lavender, comfrey and sage, herbs and vegetables for healing and eating, water pumped from a deep aquafer, clean air, mountains no matter where I look. The Lombardi's are my inspiration. This chacra a grounding place. A place my daughter will always return to because this is the hub of business for her ranches: Colopilli, Buta Mallin, and Ranquilco.

CHURCHILL DOWNS LOUISVILLE, KENTUCKY

MAY 1980

MARCH OF 1980 BROUGHT A THIRD MS ATTACK, but by this juncture, I had it dialed in. I knew the signs: extreme fatigue, cardboard feet, loss of sensation. A call to Dr. Appel in Houston brought Prednisone, bedrest, and relief within a month or two. By May I was functioning in the world again.

As much as I loved all aspects of racehorse training and breeding, I lacked the physical stamina to fully engage. My frustration was that to the casual eye, mine included, I seemed perfectly healthy. No one would ever guess I had MS, or that I'd gone through one major and two lesser bouts of paralysis. While I regained my ability to walk and normal movement patterns after these three attacks, my energy remained subpar. It could take three days or more to recover when

I over-exerted myself physically and it took so much less activity to over-exert myself. At this point, I only had one horse in training and realized it was time to turn her over to another trainer.

In addition, once Bob and I finally split, I couldn't train at Folsom. Each time I saw Bob's new girlfriend with Ginny's Little Eva, it was as if all the air in my body had been expelled with one great wallop. Thinking about how I'd lost David to Sheryl—he'd married her when I chose Bob—felt the same. All in all, thinking put me in a funk and work drew me out. I decided to focus on my art.

The National Multiple Sclerosis Society had followed up with me several times. They saw potential in the model of a successful fundraising program started in Canada with harness racing and thought a similar program could work in the United States. Given my experience in the racing world as a breeder and licensed trainer, my moneyed connections, my looks, and the fact that I had MS, they were sure I was the one to lead the campaign and generate lucrative ideas for fundraising events.

On a balmy spring Saturday, the first one in May, I sat on the edge of my sofa watching Genuine Risk win the 1980 Kentucky Derby. Genuine Risk was the first filly in sixty-five years to beat the boys; the first filly in twenty-one years to even run for the roses and only the second filly in Derby history to lift her head proud with the roses around her neck. She was so fit and sleek and proud, I just had to paint her. The fact that Sally Humphreys had bred her and Diane Firestone had trained her sealed my resolve to commemorate her as a tribute to the power of women rising in a man's world.

This idea lit a fire. The day after the race, I drove to Churchill Downs to see Genuine Risk. I sketched and snapped rolls of film, sketching and snapping until I felt I had enough material to work from. At my studio at Mother's place on the lake, I assembled my watercolors and began. Most watercolors took just hours, but I was so meticulous with this painting that it took me a week. During that week, while I painted, I came up with the idea of a limited-edition print series to sell with half the net proceeds going to The National Multiple Sclerosis Society. But I needed to get the word out. I didn't want to offer up some drop-in-the-bucket donation. I knew the money could be big with the right exposure.

NEW ORLEANS, LOUISIANA

1980

THE HORSES' BENEVOLENT AND PROTECTIVE AGENCY (HPBA) was the go-to organization for thoroughbreds and jockeys who had been hurt and needed help. HPBA published a monthly national magazine called *The Horseman's Journal*. Jack Defee, HPBA's president, lived and worked in New Orleans. Over the years we had become good friends through our racing ties. Jack was aware of the profiles on me that had recently appeared in other national publications such as *The New York Times* and *McCall's*. He knew my record as a trainer and was mindful and empathetic about my battle with MS. When I pitched my idea, coupled with splitting the net proceeds with The National Multiple Sclerosis Society, Jack said, "Well, in that case, *The Horseman's Journal* will donate a page to promote it."

My excitement about the Genuine Risk painting exceeded anything I'd done in a while. I titled the print series, "For More Than Roses." For

More Than Roses because this filly ran not for money or glory, but because she was born to run. What set her apart was that she had the heart to reach beyond her normal capacity. Reaching beyond is what makes life worth living. In those efforts to fundraise for a disease that to this day still has no cure, I wanted to reach out to those afflicted, to motivate and demonstrate that no matter the obstacle, don't quit. Stretch a bit more . . . with all your heart.

I dragged my sister, Sandra, along to the printers to proof the print on the press. This allowed me control of the colors of the four-color separations, making sure they were true before the final run.

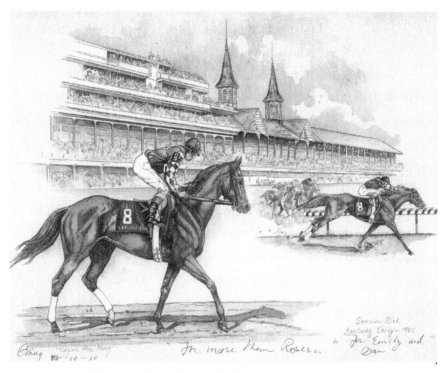

IN 1980, I PAINTED THIS WATERCOLOR OF GENUINE RISK AT CHURCHILL DOWNS IN LOUISVILLE, KENTUCKY. TITLED "FOR MORE THAN ROSES", PRINTS WERE SOLD TO BENEFIT THE NATIONAL MS SOCIETY.

The result exceeded my expectations. I was too jazzed to settle in at my twelve-foot trailer on a friend's farm in Folsom where I'd been living since my breakup with Bob. Instead, I pointed the car to Uptown New Orleans and our favorite oyster bar.

Walking through the door, I literally bumped into the back of a man. Very elegant. Cashmere jacket, sleek black BMW still idling at the curb, dark hair graying slightly at the temples.

Distracted with the hostess, he glanced over his shoulder in the most cursory way and said, "Excuse me," at the same instant I did. A fraction of a second later he turned fully toward me and asked, "May I buy you some oysters?"

Richard Allen Brunswick, M.D. or Dick, as I came to know him, was a pediatric cardiovascular thoracic heart surgeon. Brilliant and dedicated, he'd sit through nights with babies he'd operated on until he knew they were stable. He taught and operated at Tulane University's School of Medicine and at New Orleans' Charity hospital. If families were unable to afford surgery, Dick would often waive his fee.

Dick had an Uptown mansion on Walnut Street, adjacent to Audubon Park. That first night after the three of us had a leisurely dinner, Dick took us on a tour of his home. Hand-painted Limoges china trimmed in gold. Waterford crystal glasses—water, red wine, white wine, champagne, liquor—enough for twenty-four full-place settings. Baby grand piano. Jean-Baptiste-Camille Corot paintings on the walls—originals. I caught Sandra's eye and we each hid a short laugh, knowing what the other's thinking—nothing wrong with a good-looking, single man with money.

Jack Defee not only donated the page for the add, but sent staff-writer Kay Coyte from *The Horseman's Journal* to interview me in New Orleans. The published piece was a four-color, five-page write-up and my launch into fame.

A month later, F. Lee Wendell, a board member of The National Multiple Sclerosis Society, who was smitten with horses and racing, had me on the phone. He had seen *The Horseman's Journal* article and wanted to thank me personally for my fundraising efforts and let me know of the tremendous opportunity to magnify those efforts by joining my creative force and spunk with The National Multiple Sclerosis Society. The society would pay all my office and travel expenses and offer advertising and assistants to coordinate fundraising using racetracks and their facilities for sponsored events—black-tie dinners, auctions, lunches, dances and, of course, races. Lee had been talking with the harness-racing people in Canada about their program. He thought it was time to bring that idea home, not only to raise money for MS, but to revive the flagging horserace industry he so loved. Lee was certain I was the person who could pull it all together, so The Race for MS was born.

I was named Chairwoman of The Race for MS and, as first years often go, we were slow out of the gate. In 1981, our second year, we brought Bill Shoemaker aboard as co-chair. He had just won the inaugural Arlington-Million race and his fame, coupled with the resources of The National Multiple Sclerosis Society, catapulted interest and attendance at events. Once we hit our stride, we made hundreds of thousands of dollars a year, eventually adding up to several million between 1980 and 1987. The concept was a win-win. Racetracks received increasing and positive exposure, thereby bringing in new spectators, which in turn filled the stands and increased revenue. Sponsors—AT&T, Merrill Lynch, Seagram's Distillery, Cartier, Rolex amongst others—received great public relations and tax deductions for their donations.

Dick and I began to date. I always met him in a bar or restaurant, usually somewhere in the French Quarter or Uptown near his home. I didn't want him to know I lived in a trailer. Dick was reserved, soft-spoken, always gentlemanly and unlike many men, deferred the conversation to me, my interests and passions. Over many leisurely dinners, Dick began to open. His mother, Rona, was one of Abe Bronfman's daughters. Abe was one of the founders of Seagram's Distillery during the Prohibition. With his intelligence and work ethic, Dick could have easily have found a place in the Seagram's empire or he could have coasted, living a life of leisure.

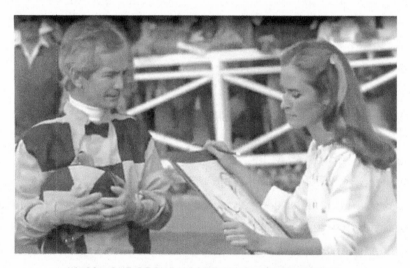

IN 1981, ONE OF THE MOST FAMOUS JOCKEYS OF ALL TIME, WILLIE SHOEMAKER (BILL TO ME), CO-CHAIRED WITH ME "THE RACE AGAINST MS." HERE WE ARE AT SANTA ANITA RACETRACK IN SOUTHERN CALIFORNIA, DOING OUR PART IN A COMMERCIAL FOR THE NATIONAL MULTIPLE SCLEROSIS SOCIETY.

Dick had everything: money, a prestigious career in a profession where he literally saved lives, good looks, humility and charm.

Everything, except love. No one, family included, had *ever* thrown him a birthday party until I came along. Margaret and Billy, his caretaking couple, took care of his day-to-day needs, but that was no substitute for love.

Within weeks of that first dinner at the oyster bar, Dick and I were snatching time together or talking on the phone nearly every day. Dick was so genuine. I felt I'd known him for a lifetime. Loving him was easy, but I was always quick to fall in love. In the short year since Bob Levi, there had been Sam, the geophysicist who lived next door to Mother, and a brief long-distance relationship with my friend Jim from Hyde Park, Maryland. Jim and another friend had gone in on a racehorse with me with the understanding that my ante in the deal was the training. The racehorse was Jim's excuse to fly down to New Orleans, bet the ponies and party. We did.

However, that all went sideways when MS sapped my strength and I had to relinquish my role as trainer. My partners were bitter about the money spent having to pay another trainer. That was the end of Jim.

Another paralysis. My third. At the time, I thought, *when will this stop?* The irony being that *I* needed to settle and stop. That therapist who had said I'd be dead at fifty-two had been right in that respect. My life was too complicated. Instead of pausing to evaluate my options and make informed decisions, I galloped off course in too many directions at once. Paralysis was my body's way of saying, *Stop. Think.* But my mind just wasn't getting the message.

I holed up in my twelve-foot trailer in Folsom with my Dalmatian, Secretariat—went to bed and stopped returning Dick's calls. After a few weeks of being put off, Dick asked around and found me. I'd been unable to cook and even if I had, would have been hard-pressed to feed myself given the partial paralysis of both hands. I was five-foot-five and down to 104 pounds. Dick stood inside the door, taking in the cramped clutter and chaos and said, "Jewish princesses shouldn't live like this." He scooped me in his arms, deposited me on the front seat of his Rolls Royce and drove me to his Uptown mansion in New Orleans where I remained off-and-on for six years.

Off-and-on being the operative condition. I became a nomad, though not completely altruistic. I crafted my nomadic lifestyle primarily to escape the heat. By my third paralysis, I had begun to notice a pattern—when the heat index in New Orleans rose into the 90s and 100s with its suffocating humidity, I wilted. And I don't mean Scarlet O'Hara back-of-the-wrist-on-the-forehead-weak-at-the-knees kind of wilt. I mean by the heat-of-the-day, I would be completely enervated, with my limbs moving as if through a trough of setting cement. I couldn't think or focus or move. All I could do was lie down. Be still.

As an ambassador for MS through The National Multiple Sclerosis Society, I had free reign over my work schedule, as well as my travel and where events were to be held. I chose strategically. New Orleans in the winter and early spring. Lexington, Kentucky and Keeneland with its pink and white dogwoods mid-spring to early summer. Iowa, to my sister Susie's farm, whenever a MS attack rendered me helpless. By the early 80s, she was married to a budding attorney and was a registered nurse. Susie instinctively seemed to know how to nurture me, prop me back up, then as gently as she had received me, reluctantly watch me hurl myself back into the world again.

Iowa often led to Chicago. From there turn right to Saratoga Springs in New York, where then president of the Saratoga Polo Club, Hal Chafee helped me raise funds, or left to Northern California and San Francisco's Bay Meadows where the weather suited me, but the racing and fundraising were not so lucrative as Saratoga. Del Mar and Santa Anita in Southern California drew better horses and clientele with deeper pockets.

During my initial fundraising years with MS, I traveled the country in my VW Vanagon camper with Secretariat, or Spot as he became known. Spot had seen me through my trials with Bob Levi and David and during my first MS paralysis. When I was completely paralyzed for three months, he kept vigil, curled at the foot of my bed. Throughout 1980 - 1987, I continued my relapse-remission cycle of MS every nine months to a year. High levels of stress, plus heat, seemed to guarantee a relapse. A trip to Susie's in Iowa surrounded by farmland, quiet, and the steady loving presence of my sister and her family seemed to guarantee remission. Often by the time I landed at Susie's I was in bad shape—physically depleted, fatigued, depressed and failing fast. It was at the farm that I began to notice that my attitude correlated with the speed with which I recovered. When I hung out lamenting my losses, my paralysis and fatigue drug on. I came to the conclusion that when I'm not happy, I don't get well.

Concurrent with my role as ambassador for The National Multiple Sclerosis Society, I was producing equine art on commission, usually

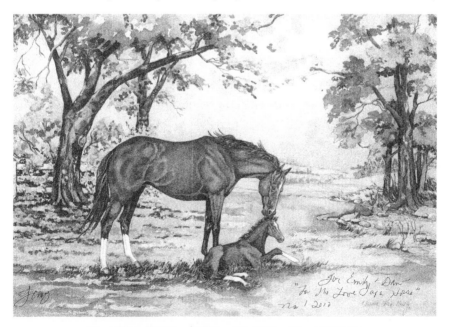

IN 1982, AFTER BEING DELAYED BY ANOTHER MS ATTACK, I COMPLETED THIS MIXED MEDIA WATERCOLOR THAT COMMEMORATED JIM BEAM'S SPONSORSHIP OF HORSE RACING. TITLED, "FOR THE LOVE OF A HORSE." LATER IT BECAME A SCULPTED BOURBON DECANTER.

for racehorse owners, sometimes for a track. Always the money behind the commission was big. In late 1979, I received a lucrative job from the president of Pan-American Life Insurance in New Orleans, Wallace B. Schmitz, to paint his Folsom farm and several of his racehorses, but I went into a paralysis. My hands didn't work. The commission was graciously deferred rather than cancelled.

In the spring of 1982, Jim Beam Distillery commissioned a sculpture to commemorate the $150,000 Jim Beam Spiral Stakes at Latonia Race Course in Florence, Kentucky. The sculpted decanter and limited-edition print titled, 'For the Love of a Horse,' show a mare standing over her newborn foal, urging it to stand, and the foal with head lifted and one foreleg bent, ready to meet the world.

Later in 1982, after meeting Lord James Crichton-Stuart at a National Multiple Sclerosis Society function in New Orleans, Lord Crichton-Stuart invited me to participate on behalf of the U.S. National Multiple Sclerosis Society. A match race at Ascot pitted master European jockey Lester Piggott against premier American jockey Bill Shoemaker in a showdown to raise 350,000 pounds for The Multiple Sclerosis International Federation. Presenting Bill with the trophy was a proud moment.

In a live follow-up interview on BBC Television with Julian Wilson, he asked how my filly Last Time Up had come to her name. With a straight face, I launched into the story of how her sire Porterhouse, covered the mare, then dropped dead. His last time up, indeed. After the interview, when I walked into the clubhouse bar, the Lord and Lady punters stood, raised their glasses and in a shout out said, "You are the toast of England."

LAKE VISTA, LOUISIANA

1982

WHILE MY LIFE AS AN ARTIST AND AMBASSADOR for MS was spinning me out of control in a delightful swept-up and heady kind of way, my relationship with Dick, solid and steadfast in all things emotional, helped keep the wheels on the cart. However, across town at Mother's Lake Vista home, the cart wobbled fiercely and was headed for the ditch. Mother was still living there when she wasn't "on vacation" at the institution. Fairly stable since her move to New Orleans, she was perking along fine until my paralyzed brother Bill moved himself, his wife and their two adopted, wild, and disabled children in with her because, as she said with a dramatic sweep of her hand, "I have all the room in the world."

What there wasn't room for was more craziness. Mother had recently been found, more than once, in her pajamas, prancing down the streets of her tidy, proper, lakefront neighborhood asking whomever she encountered, always men, whether they'd like a role in the play she was writing.

At home, Bill's wife, in an effort to control the uncontrollable behavior of their two wild children, tied them to kitchen chairs for an hour at a crack, while Mother paced and chain-smoked and mumbled. I happened upon this scene one day after I'd received a nearly incomprehensible call from her. The house was an asylum.

Off Mother went on another vacation, which seemed the right course of action, until the day I visited and found her in a straight-jacket. Take it from me, you never want to see your mother in a locked ward or find her in a straight-jacket. Both are traumatizing.

In an effort to help preserve Mother's remaining sanity and money, Sandra, Susie and I uprooted and replanted her in Susie's basement apartment in the farmhouse in Iowa. Pleased with ourselves at having done the right thing, we thought Susie's stable, Leave-It-to-Beaver family life would be just the salve after the drama of living with Bill and his family. Our relief was short-lived.

Mother hated Susie's. She was mean to the grandchildren, chased off the hired help, and was driving Susie nuts while at the same time breaking her heart.

Maybe she needed to be with people her own age. We checked her into a nice nursing home, the kind that doesn't smell like disinfectant and pee, the kind where residents decorate their own rooms and there are fresh flowers in all the communal areas and the food tastes like food. Mother hated the nursing home. She couldn't smoke in her room and she'd smoked since she was eighteen. After packing her bags, Mother slipped on her jacket and flipped a lit match into her waste basket before strolling to the front desk to ask them to call her a taxi. On her way out the door she said, "Oh, you might want to check my room. There seems to be a fire."

With that swansong, Mother finally got what she wanted and moved in with Sandra in Chicago.

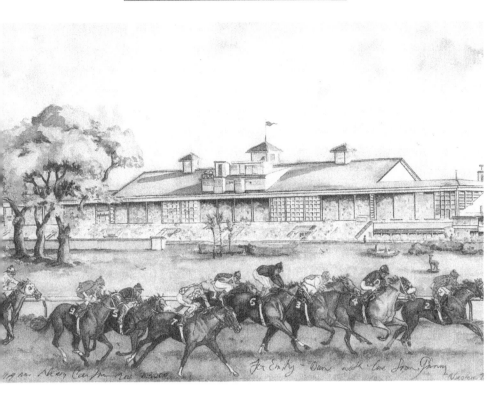

TITLED "NEW ORLEANS FAIRGROUNDS", I
PAINTED THIS WATERCOLOR WHILE IN NEW
ORLEANS, LOUISIANA IN 1983.

NEW ORLEANS, LOUISIANA

1984

BY 1984 AND 1985, THE PRESIDENT of the Saratoga Springs Polo Club had dubbed me the "Jet Gypsy." My beloved VW Vanagon camper and Spot were parked at Susie's in Iowa. With thirteen major events spanning those years, I flew. In between, I worked the phones five days a week creating, coordinating, and inspiring staff and volunteers alike to pony up their time and talent; vendors to consider discounted fees for services; the moneyed to donate gifts for auction and to sponsor tables at events for their racing friends and family.

By 1985, Dick and I had been drifting in our relationship. I knew I wanted him. He and I had been through the time of marriage, no-marriage, me insisting we could work things out, Dick not so sure. And always, the initial warmth of coming together again after I'd been out of town for weeks or months kept some level of hope alive in both of us.

That year, with Dick's help and my racehorse earnings, I bought five-acres in the farmlands of Folsom and built a small Cajun cottage. Dick was happy to see me become more independent. I moved in just before hurricane season. My neighbor across the lane, Dorsey, was my age, tall, with a striking head of sun-streaked hair, a swimmer with a pool. He was a psychiatrist and practicing neurologist at a hospital he owned in Covington. We began to date. I was completely honest with Dick.

Shortly after I moved into my cottage, the forecast one early morning was for a hurricane. I taped my windows, filled water jugs for myself and Spot, put the transistor radio in the bathroom where Spot and I planned to wait out the storm in the tub. Dick called, concerned, wanting me to come to town, but it was too late to make the drive. The storm was blowing in. Dorsey called from across the lane and invited me to weather the storm at his house. Spot and I ran over without a second thought. Dorsey's brilliant blue eyes took me in in a way that I hadn't been seen in a long time, while outside the winds howled and trees bent low.

In the storm's aftermath, I had a lover and a case of guilt. I debated calling Dick, but he beat me to it. Even though we had both accepted the quiet end of our intimate relationship two years prior, we were still unraveling our long-term liaison. That we loved each other complicated the issue. Dick wanted me in is life, but not as wife or even live-in partner. When I told him about Dorsey, how I'd never intended to sleep with him, but how I was swept away, Dick said, "I'll never love anyone more than you. But you have needs I can't meet. I can't marry you, but I'll *always* be here for you."

Heartbroken at Dick's final resolve, it was time for me to find someone else to love and marry. Maybe Dorsey. But two days later, Dorsey's girlfriend called. To compare notes.

My health began a rapid decline. It was so hot and humid in Folsom that the air-conditioning couldn't keep up with the heat index.

I couldn't get out of bed and when I did it was to drag myself to the bathroom. I remember lurching footboard to doorframe and stopping to brace myself, arms straight, elbows locked, on the sink counter to rest. In the mirror, I saw the sun-streaked hair; fine Patrician bones; straight and even nose; the eyes golden-brown, searching, then casting to the horoscope I'd taped to the mirror a few weeks before: *Have hope. Love will soon enter your life.* From where I stood, that didn't seem possible. Nothing did. I was alone with Spot and it wasn't enough.

One afternoon, exhausted from the heat, the paralysis, all of it, I decided to take a large dose of sleeping pills. I thought sleeping uninterrupted for a few days might bring me back. When I came to, more than twenty-four hours later, still drug-stupid, I thought, "Shit. I could have killed myself." I called my girlhood friend, Janice. She had just moved to Rifle, Colorado. She and her husband, Ron, came to get me, Spot and my VW Vanagon. There in the Rocky Mountain cool, in the loving care of my dearest friend, I rested and recovered once again.

ASPEN, COLORADO

1986

ONCE I FELT BETTER, I HAD TO GO FIND some horses to ride. While I could no longer gallop and exercise racehorses, milder, gentler gaits on calmer steeds was therapeutic. A woman I'd known in New Orleans, Bonnie Corner, had told me she was on her way to Aspen to train polo ponies, so one bright morning, I kissed Janice on the forehead, hopped into my VW Vanagon with Spot and headed to Aspen.

Aspen was small, and it didn't take but two inquiries to get pointed to Crystal Island Ranch where Bonnie supposedly worked. What land! Three-thousand acres with a river tumbling through and three cabins with a private lake and spectacular view of Mt. Sopris. At the first cabin, caretakers directed me to a larger log cabin. When the door opened, my stomach lurched and my heart came to a standstill before it began to gallop. The man before me was tall, well- built, and trim. He dressed simply—classic white shirt tucked into Levis and deep-brown, handmade leather boots. His auburn hair was wavy, tousled, reflecting the playfulness of his smile. Bright blue inquisitive eyes held me with bemused interest as I stood somewhat slack-jawed.

This was the man I'd waited for all my life.

I forgot everything. My name, my family's insanity, suicide, paralysis, MS. The only moment was the one I stood in. "Umm," I finally sputtered out. I could feel the heat creeping up my neck into my cheeks. "I'm looking for Bonnie Corner. Does she work here?"

"No," he said. A whole world in those eyes balanced in good measure with that dazzling smile. "But I bet we can find her at the polo field." He peered over my shoulder to the idling camper van with Spot sitting shotgun in the passenger seat. "Put on your jeans and boots and you can be my groom."

I followed his old classic Mercedes to the ranch's polo field. Bonnie caught sight of the VW Vanagon with Spot sitting tall and sprinted to greet us. I was so glad to see a familiar face. Plus, connecting with Bonnie gave me an out on walking hot-walking horses in the midday heat.

It turned out the man I'd waited for all my life was none other than the owner of Crystal Island Ranch, Ashley Carrithers. At half-time in the polo match, he sauntered over, shirtless, sweat beaded on his chest. My legs felt weak, as they'd often felt during an MS attack, but this paralysis was different. It originated in my solar plexus. Magnetic. Like when two strong magnets come within range of each other, there's the point at which they can no longer be kept apart. That night Ashley invited me to camp at his lake. We had dinner at the cabin where I met the product of his first marriage, his fourteen-year-old son, T.A., whom I thought might be deaf and dumb as he didn't say one word the entire evening.

My attraction to Ashley scared me. Something deep warned that if I let myself get too close, he'd consume me, so I initially refused his advances. Worried he'd bolt, I didn't tell him I had MS for about ten days. When I did, he laughed and said, "Well, I never did like anyone normal." But behind that easy acceptance, there wasn't an inkling of what MS was or what an attack could do. He took me at face value. I looked fine, therefore, I was fine. Why complicate the uncomplicated?

Not being my first time up, I rode this one a bit more cautiously than I had with Bob Levi or Dick Brunswick. I knew better than to live with him. I realized in order to maintain my health and not go into an MS relapse, I needed to conserve my energy. I needed rest to appear light, vibrant, healthy. I rented a place on the Crystal River in Carbondale, about thirty-minutes from Crystal Island Ranch. I rested every other day—one day and night with Ashley and the next day in bed in my apartment. Next, to ensure I'd see Ashley daily, I bought an Arabian named Karma, the son of Shah el Shalim, the Arabian white stallion Ashley rode daily during his ranch work. I boarded Karma at the ranch, where I had continuous access not only to Ashley, but to one of the most beautiful ranches I'd ever seen.

I knew what I wanted and I knew what I had to do to get it. Ashley, for all his worldly experience and good looks was still quite naïve and trusting.

Like all good deals, there were a few hitches, the first being Ashley's friend Nancy, a single Aspen socialite who'd talked Ashley into siring her child. Nancy's pitch was, "It's you, Michael Douglas, or the sperm bank in Denver." Ashley, always obliging, complied. Had the deal ended there, my mind would have eased. However, Nancy called at night, wanting to bring baby Juliana by or bring her rich and famous friends to the lake for the day. What most concerned me was that Nancy and Ashley were headed to Africa in a few months to spend a full moon with Kuki Gallmann, who wrote, *I Dreamed of Africa*. I dreamed Nancy and Juliana would mysteriously vanish before Ashley swept off to Africa with them.

Another hitch was the money. Where Ashley's came from was a mystery. Over time, conversation yielded that he had never done any business for himself. Ashley was a visionary, not the generative type. This nagged uncomfortably in the far recesses of my mind. I'd known lots of moneyed men. In my lexicon, there had been several types— those who worked like Bob Levi (albeit his work was below-board with the mob), the silver-spooners who'd had it handed to them in a tidy trust fund at the ripe old age of twenty-five, and hybrids like Dick who had all the money he'd ever need, but chose to work his passion as a pediatric heart surgeon.

Ashley was connected. The rich and famous were a familiar sight at Crystal Island's private lake. With Hollywood friends, he talked about making a movie. He owned a 100,000-acre estancia, or ranch, in Northern Patagonia, along with Crystal Island's 3000 acres. He also had land in Northern California. Bought in reaction to the Vietnam War, he and some Duke University buddies ponied up and started the hippie commune, NOTA (None Of The Above). Ashley founded Island Foundation Press, which is one of the most respected non-profit environmental presses in the world, as well as Island Foundation, which took part in the formation of the Conservation Easement which has saved millions of acres in the U.S. from development.

Over time I found out the money came from his second wife, Cathy, daughter of a billionaire. Ashley had become a polo-playing philanthropist and land baron through his legal bond with her money.

Money was not new to me. Both my parents had come from landed families and as a psychiatrist, my father had provided a large home on San Souci Island in Waterloo, Iowa, complete with motorboat docked off the lower garden for summer weekend fun. Mother had daily help with cooking, washing, cleaning. I had a horse and a place to ride it.

The horsey set with whom I rubbed elbows in New Orleans and Kentucky had led to my work with The National Multiple Sclerosis Society. Our successful fundraising campaign, The Race Against MS, with Bill Shoemaker, thrust me into news and television notoriety on a national level. Meeting Lord James Crichton-Stuart in 1982 and my attendance at Ascot had swung open the selective and exclusive door to Saratoga Springs in New York. Saratoga Springs was the pinnacle of the U.S. horseracing world. To be embraced by that company as a trainer, breeder, equine artist and minor celebrity fundraiser, gave me occasional access to yachts, Lear jets, and privileges otherwise withheld. Initially wide-eyed in a deer-in-the-headlights sort of way, I learned to adapt to the demands of the moment, giving the casual onlooker the impression I was born to this life.

Ashley left me wide-eyed in a different sort of way. At Crystal Island Ranch at the foot of Mt. Sopris with its polo field, private lake, and cabin rather than mansion, I felt I'd found home. More than that, his world, while privileged and moneyed, lacked the ostentatiousness of the New York crowd. As did Ashley. I once asked what his true ambition was and he said, "To study metaphysics."

NEW YORK CITY, NEW YORK

OCTOBER 1986

AT THE END OF SEPTEMBER, ASHLEY flew off to Africa with Nancy and Juliana as scheduled. Imagining him in Nancy's presence day-in and day-out left me frazzled. Ashley and I did have plans to travel to Argentina in late November, to Estancia Ranquilco, but that still left Nancy and Juliana with a lot of time to win him over.

In Carbondale, Ashley was never far from my mind, but I didn't have time to sit around pining. I had a big meeting in New York with The National Multiple Sclerosis Society where I planned to submit my resignation as Chairwoman for The Race Against MS. The bottom line with MS was that I never knew when my body would stop functioning and I'd be unable to provide for myself.

I'd decided to focus what energy I had on my equine art and Ashley.

It so happened Dick Brunswick was in town too. I'd kept Dick posted on my move to Carbondale and of the life I'd created around Ashley. Dick was happy for me in a sad sort of way. He wanted the best for me, even if he wasn't the one to provide it.

Over a New York dinner one balmy evening, he reached across the table and took my hand. Sleepy from the meal and wine, my mind snapped to as Dick told me of his plan to pass some of his inheritance on to me. He said the half-million dollars was money he'd never need and that his mother, Rona Bronfman, had even agreed to pay the inheritance tax for me as she would have for him.

This was a new view from the top. I was thirty-seven. Ready to be married. Ready to be my own woman. Ready for the insecurity and worry and struggle of making a living between bouts of MS paralysis to end. And here was Dick, open-heartedly handing me a half-million dollars with no strings attached. "I just want you to feel secure," he said. This changed everything and nothing. Everything in that I could now support myself. I could go to Ashley, if not as financial equal, then as a woman solid in my own financial standing. Nothing, in that this money would not change my pursuit of Ashley. I suspected Dick hoped it might.

Dick said he'd done a background check on Ashley Carrithers and some of what he'd found worried him. Ashley took large financial risks, leveraging those risks in precarious ways, but so far had not come to much harm, given that he was still coasting on his divorce settlement. "Also," Dick said, looking away toward the clatter at the bar, "Ashley's quite the ladies' man."

The following morning brought my meeting with The National Multiple Sclerosis Society. They accepted my resignation with regret, but understood. I had been volunteering for MS since 1980 and given the progression of my disease, the need to reduce stress and conserve energy was paramount. I also informed them I'd be out of the country in Argentina for an indefinite period. The board not only thanked me for my years of tireless service, but informed me that I'd been nominated for a Patient Achievement Award in the coming year. The National Multiple Sclerosis Society did have one request—travel to Belmont Race Track to film a segment about the work I'd done for the Race Against MS.

When I returned home to Colorado after New York and filming at Belmont, I was sagging. I'd had no word from Ashley on my trip and the uncertainty as to where I stood versus Nancy, combined with the stress of travel and filming, had frayed me. A letter from Africa lifted my spirits. It was brief, but all I needed. "I'm cutting the trip short. I just can't be with this woman any longer. Coming home soon." He'd signed it, *With love.*

By the time Ashley returned, the chill of late fall had settled at Crystal Island Ranch. The first snow had capped the Rockies. Canadian geese were still migrating south. They'd overnight at Ashley's lake, then in the morning rise with a great honking clamor, circling until all gathered, then they'd line themselves up in their V-formations and follow the force of their instinct south.

ESTANCIA RANQUILCO, NORTHERN PATAGONIA, ARGENTINA

NOVEMBER 1986

HOW WISE OF ASHLEY TO GO SOUTH with the geese. Ashley had been migrating for years to the southern hemisphere and Northern Patagonia. The ranch, Estancia Ranquilco, really was 100,000 acres. The other property, Lago Lolog, just outside of San Martin de los Andes was eighty acres.

His ex-wife's money had paid for it all, including Crystal Island Ranch. Hearsay was every property Ashley owned, except for NOTA and Lago Lolog had two essentials—an airstrip and a polo field. That led to rumors of drug running and money laundering, which Dick's research failed to prove out.

Stepping off the plane into the brilliant warmth and sun of Buenos

Aires felt like coming home, but home was still cross-country, nearly to Chile. Our next flight ferried us to San Martin de los Andes and from there, Ashley flew us into Estancia Ranquilco in his Cessna 172 taildragger. As Ashley's family was in residence, separate bedrooms were the plan, however, that's not how it turned out. I met his parents, Charlie and Dossie, and his sister, Annie, at dinner that first night. All very formal. We dressed for dinner at ten, served on Wedgewood china, with silver and crystal.

Dinner started festive enough. As Patron, Ashley headed the table. His younger sister, Annie, had been acting Patrona since Ashley's ex-wife's departure. I sat to Ashley's right across from Dossie, while Charlie was seated next to her. Charlie was a bit of a stiff stick. Harvard. Retired banker. Full head of silver-grey hair, pipe a permanent fixture unless he was sipping a stiff one or eating. Walked with a staff. The overall effect was Hemmingwayesque. Dossie on the other hand, was everything a girl might want in a mother-in-law. Scripps University in Southern California. Loved a good cocktail and story, preferably together, and had been a stay-at-home mom.

Annie sat, tall and imperious, at the head of the table with a little silver bell at her right hand to ring the kitchen help to clear and bring in the next course. She was a chef in her own right and clearly took pride in her role as Patrona and ran Ranquilco accordingly. She tracked pantry contents, liquor stores, and the daily where, when and what of staff with a civil formality. She made it clear her orders would not be tampered with.

If not for Dossie's light-hearted chatter and social agility, the evening would never have gotten off the ground. Annie was stiff, issuing short, succinct answers to my questions, volunteering nothing. By the second of five courses, Charlie had begun a launch of verbal arrows at Dossie's every comment. I had no idea how she withstood his ridicule. It hurt my heart, yet Dossie just laughed and had another glass of wine. Ashley seemed impervious to it all.

Ashley had first come to Argentina for the fly fishing. He arrived with a fancy bamboo rod, worn-through blue jeans, chambray shirt, and tattered cowboy hat. When he found out what a dollar could buy and surveyed the expanse available for the price—lands with lakes and rivers, lands still untouched by industry and development—he stayed for the land.

The Argentine summer was magic. I had to remind myself that it was December, January, March, that friends in the northern hemisphere were shoveling snow and horses were turned out in blankets or stalled against the Colorado cold. Life here was on and of the earth. Energy was solar and turbine powered. We dined in the evenings by candlelight. Fruits and vegetables were harvested from an onsite garden; beef and sheep and goats were slaughtered as needed. Eggs gathered from coops. Water issued pure from underground springs. Wheat was ground with an old stone mill.

Eating this way, swimming in the Rio Trocoman just below the house, riding daily, painting and sketching the endless landscape and being madly in love, I began to heal in a way I never had. Deeply. My muscles regained strength I remembered from before my first MS attack, even my hands regained some of their original fine motor skills.

On the other end of the spectrum was Ashley's family. Annie, Charlie and T.A., Ashley's son, who had shown up for the month of January. All but Dossie left me with no doubt that I did not, nor would I ever, belong. Annie wanted nothing to do with my attempts to help in the kitchen or offers of friendship. Charlie continued his dinner assaults on Dossie and began aiming them in my direction. I left the table. Teenage T.A. spoke in monosyllables when he spoke at all.

By mid-March I told Ashley I was leaving. It was two weeks earlier than planned, but I'd had enough of his family and was sick of the staff's hailing and bowing to El Patron. Plus, I didn't speak any Spanish. Nada. Which left me isolated in the company of my art or Ashley or, occasionally, Dossie. I loved Ashley, but I began to feel as if I'd had too much chocolate. Ashley and I could regroup back in the states, away from his family.

Before my departure, Ashley asked me to live with him permanently when we returned to Colorado. He'd been trying to get me to move in with him since our first days together. Each time the answer was no. "The only way I'll live with you is if we're married. You have two- weeks to decide." I was still searching for the right man to marry, but there was no doubt in my mind or heart my man was Ashley.

In Colorado, the snow was still deep. I settled into my rental in Carbondale and caught up with the world, reveled in my appreciation of English and relaxed into a quiet self-sufficiency. Now that I had my strength back, I needed to decide whether to sell or rent my Cajun cottage at Folsom. It felt like lifetimes ago that I'd lived, worked, and loved in New Orleans. I called and filled Dick in on my Argentine summer and the fact that I was healthier than I'd been in years. I was in full remission. He was still concerned about Ashley's lack of business acumen and womanizing, but he also knew me well enough to know that once I got my teeth into something, I wouldn't be put off. He heard the joy in my voice and repeated his promise, "I'll *always* be here for you."

I decided to rent out the Cajun cottage, just in case.

When Ashley arrived home, it was as if he brought the Argentine sun with him. Snow melted, spring flowers began to pop up in the ranch's meadows, and we were together again in a place where his family was not, where we were on even footing because I was no longer his guest, and I understood every word.

NEW YORK CITY, NEW YORK

MARCH 30, 1987

SPRINGTIME IN CENTRAL PARK. NEW YORKERS uncharacteristically playing in the grass, laughing, running in the sun between beds lush with tulips and daffodils. Our party reflected the city's high as Sandra, Mom and I, Ashley and Dossie, and Dick checked into suites at the Carlyle Hotel, compliments of Dick. This was the first-time Ashley had met any of my family. No accident there. I'd worried the crazy might scare him off. Once Mother had moved in with Sandra in Chicago, and I'd handled evicting Bill—my quadriplegic brother and his family—from her home, I'd written the family off. No help at all. Once Mother's house sold, each of us was free of the other. No more old-money ties and manipulation of purse strings.

This trip to New York was my moment. The National Multiple

Sclerosis Society's Dinner of Champions was a black-tie affair at which I was to be honored, along with Bill Shoemaker and The New York Giants. I trusted that as long as mother was with Sandra, she would behave herself.

Sandra and Mother met Ashley for the first time in the bar at the Algonquin Hotel. Mother was on her best behavior. Bourbon in hand, she leaned forward in the club chair to admire my engagement ring—a two-carat diamond set deep into a broad gold band. It had been Ashley's grandfather's. For me the ring was an afterthought. I wasn't the kind of woman who really needed a ring.

On his return from Argentina, Ashley had said nothing about marriage for a day. I bided my time. That evening at dinner at his cabin he'd asked, "Don't you want to know what I'm giving you for your engagement present?" Relief washed through me. His gift was the grey polo-pony I'd fallen in love with in San Martin de los Andes.

By the evening of the Dinner of Champions, we'd been in New York for three days. Dick had been wining and dining my ever-growing entourage around the city. Friends had flown in from New Orleans, California, Colorado. That morning, Dick had hosted a breakfast in my honor at the Carlyle Hotel with family and friends. I'd been lifted by some invisible hand out of the mental poverty I'd been living in since my MS diagnosis to the top of the mountain. It never occurred to me for a moment to look down.

That night the ballroom overflowed with black ties and evening gowns. I wore my favorite off-white, floor-length gown with the diamond necklace and bracelet Bob Levi had given me, and my engagement ring. Following several speeches, the organizers showed a short film compiled from seven different segments of television interviews I'd done around the country over the years. The film garnered a standing ovation, as did my speech which followed. Stepping down from the stage, as I took Ashley's hand, so warm and solid in mine, I'd never felt so loved, appreciated, and deeply secure.

CRYSTAL ISLAND RANCH, COLORADO

SEPTEMBER 1987

WE MARRIED ON THE SEVENTH on the full moon in 1987. An auspicious start. The three-day extravaganza leading to our vows started on Friday night with a dance party at Andre's Discotheque with the ceiling opened to the celestial stars. Dossie, in her new-found freedom—Charlie had died in his natty old chair in a one-bedroom apartment less than a year after she'd left him—danced until her legs nearly buckled.

On Saturday, we held a huge asado (Argentine barbeque) and polo game at our field, memorable because no matter how fervently I embraced my future with Ashley, the past kept cropping up in funny little ways. Bob Levi for instance. Not that he had been invited, but neither had the woman who had usurped my place as Bob's lover and

Ginny's Little Eva's trainer. Yet there she was on our polo field. Bob had married her. Rich, pretty, horsey, healthy. She'd met all the prerequisites. Now divorced, she said she'd left Bob because he was spending too much of her money. Which is, I believe, the same reason Cathy left Ashley.

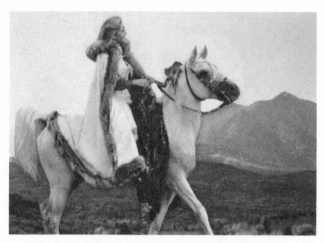

IT'S 1987 AND I'M ON MY WAY TO BECOMING MRS. ASHLEY CARRITHERS, RIDING SHAH EL SHALIM, A GIFT FROM MY SOON-TO-BE-HUSBAND. OUR WEDDING WAS AT CRYSTAL ISLAND RANCH AT THE FOOT OF MT. SOPRIS IN THE ASPEN VALLEY IN COLORADO.

Sunday, we married at the lake. George Stranahan, an ordained minister and Aspen philanthropist, and Dik Darnell, a Lakota Sioux Medicine Carrier and gifted musician, presided. I wore an emerald-green silk blouse, tucked into white elk-skin riding pants. A laced vest matching the pants peeked out from under a hooded cape lined in white satin and trimmed with Canadian lynx. Handmade, knee-high lace-up moccasins completed my ensemble. With a late-summer bouquet of wild flowers and sage, I was every bit Lakota Sioux princess, if not in blood, then by assimilation. Ashley's leather pants, braided up the front, and his emerald-green shirt matched mine. I'd had his ring styled after mine—a broad white-gold band with a deep-set sapphire— silver and gold, his favorite colors.

After the ceremony, Cristal champagne and toasts flowed, then Ashley and I rode off under the full moon on our white Arabians, Shah el Shalim and his son Karma. The reception, held at Red Stone Castle, which we'd rented in its entirety to house family and friends, ended sometime after sunrise the next morning. I had to lie down every few hours to recuperate, but nothing could stop me from dancing.

With little time to come down from our wedding, we launched into the honeymoon with Ashley's boyhood friend Walter Sedgwick, known as Sedg, and his wife. We boarded the train in Vancouver, B.C. for a two-day trip across Canada, our eventual destination the eastern part of the country where the Sedgwick's had a rustic summer cottage on a lake.

Sedg and Ashley had grown up together in Gates Mill, Ohio, a wealthy suburb of Cleveland. Sedg's family was blue-blooded as they come, while Ashley's was more up and coming. Sedg and his wife occasionally resided in their family home in Thomasville, Georgia on Mill Pond Plantation—a sprawling 10,000-acre quail-hunting retreat. The main house was a rambling mansion, with ancient Live Oaks dripping moss from their branches. Black help ran the home and attended to family and guest needs. A black man drove the horse-drawn wagon carrying hunters with shotguns in the crooks of bent elbows, while the hunting dogs raced ahead, flushing quail. A cinematic scene straight out of the old South.

On the train, we had first-class sleeping cabins; a first-class lounge car, complete with bar; and reservations for dinner each night in the dining car. I anticipated the trip as a time to relax and let down after the non-stop excitement and activity around our wedding. I hadn't realized how tired I was until I'd sat for a few hours watching the Canadian wilderness slip by. After about eight hours of constant rocking, I remembered a car trip I'd taken from Chicago to Florida. How the constant movement had induced a MS relapse, complete with paralysis, and I panicked.

"Ashley, I have to get off this train."

"Impossible."

I had never spoken to Ashley in any depth about my MS symptoms and the consequences of ignoring them. He'd never seemed all that interested or concerned. He knew I had MS. I'd told him within the first few weeks of our dating. I had to, because I couldn't keep up with him. But because he'd never seen me in a relapse, he had no respect for how I needed to listen to my body and let it dictate my schedule and activity. Ashley, with his strapping good health and avidly adventurous mind, thought it ludicrous to let anything other than schedule and time run the show.

"I'm getting off at the next stop. I'll meet up with you." Even after I related the story about the car trip and its adverse effects, Ashley said, "Don't be ridiculous, Ginny."

In the end, I didn't get off the train. Instead, I took some tranquilizers and curled up in my berth. I had averted a relapse with the use of minor tranquilizers. The trick was to recognize anxiety immediately and reduce it. During the years I'd been with Bob Levi, I'd practiced Transcendental Meditation. It worked if practiced regularly, but nothing had been regular about the past seven years of my life.

EL HEUCÚ, NORTHERN PATAGONIA, ARGENTINA

APRIL 2, 2017

MY DAYS ARE PREDICTABLE, YET not predictable. While my body vegetates in this partially paralyzed stasis—my legs no longer work; I'm incontinent; I'm unable to sit up on my own—my mind works perfectly fine. Well, fine if I don't try to remember details too far back. I'm certain the sclerosis on my brain has increased. It causes me to slur which makes me sound more out of it than I am. But I know what's going on. I know who lies, who cheats, who steals. I know more than people think I know and sometimes that works to my advantage.

My main caregiver, Rosa, has been out for a month with gallstones and other gastrointestinal issues that required surgery and a long recovery. As my caregivers are required to support my weight as they transfer me from bed to wheelchair, a strong back and core muscles are essential. I miss Rosa. She helps with my art. Even though all but the index finger and thumb on my right hand are permanently curled into the palm, I can use my left hand to make ceramic-tiled trays.

With much assistance, assistance Rosa enjoys providing, I can also work on the wall mural in the pool house. As time goes by, the painting on it becomes more abstract. I used to swim too. I used to stand up 100 times a day, hanging onto a sturdy metal gate outside. I used to imagine myself walking with a walker again. Now, my muscles are so weak, I'm lucky if I stand ten times. I used to be so determined, but somehow determination has slipped away and in its place, I find complacency and the need to find fault. Mostly with the food, since food is one of my main pleasures.

I want to tell you about the food. Or really, about the cook. M comes three-hours a day, Monday through Friday, from nine to noon. She had been with us for seven years—five-and-a-half of those years "in black" and one-and-a-half "in white." "In the black" means an employee is working under the radar. If someone collects a government pension for a disability, it's against the law for them to work. Most people in El Heucú collect a government pension for something. Yet the ones who can find employment on the side work in the black. Double-dipping. "In the white" means an employee is working for you legally and certain benefits must be supplied under certain conditions. The government has a list of regulations as long as your leg, and if an employer does not follow them, they can be sued. Being a socialist-based system, the employee usually prevails.

Ten months ago, M gave birth to another son. She already has two at home. Because she was in white, we paid her entire salary for her six-month maternity leave. Upon her return to work, she appealed to Sky to have one of her older sons bring the baby to her when it was time to nurse. Being a nursing mother herself, Sky gave her the go-ahead.

In the past two months, M's cooking has become progressively unimaginative, oily and salty. Even though I ask for less salt, she never complies. Lunch is our main meal of the day. Often, she is too lazy to walk to the garden and pick tomatoes, carrots, chard, or kale for a simple salad, or if she does, she picks lettuce and nothing more. The time her baby is here has increased to an hour or more a day. From all reports M works roughly an hour to an hour-and-a-half on her best days.

She has grown surly. We are sure she is trying to get fired. If we fire her, we must pay her full salary for the entire time she's been in the white, plus two-months additional salary. The whole situation puts me in a mood and moods are not conducive to my physical health.

Sky and Leo are here. Sky's presence at the chacra incites the whole town to turn out. All right, I exaggerate, but the coming and going is excessive when Sky rolls in. A man was here last night at nine-thirty to be paid for materials he sells and delivers to the ranch. A few weeks ago, a man came asking for payment for goats that Sky's half-brother, T.A., had bought several months prior. Of course, Sky paid him. She can't afford not to.

I don't know why I'm telling you all this. Perhaps because I'm very social and you speak English. Try being social in a language you speak marginally with people you have nothing in common with. It's tough. That's why I depend so much on Sky. My sun rises and sets by Sky and Leo. I didn't have her until I was thirty-nine. I'd had MS for twelve-years by then. Having her was a conscious decision. I promised the creator that if I were granted a child, I'd dedicate my life to her. I did. In turn, Sky now cares for me. I never meant for her to be my keeper. But this is what it has come to and I am grateful. I wish the responsibility for Ranquilco's livestock, Leo, and my welfare had not coincided so squarely. She's simultaneously pulled in each direction. At twenty-eight, strong and supple, she bends like the poplars in our fierce Patagonia winds. But I worry that these trials are just the prelude to some unprecedented hundred-year storm.

GULF OF MEXICO

OCTOBER 1987

A TREASURE HUNT? WHY NOT? The honeymoon over, Ashley and I made a pit stop at Crystal Island Ranch to exchange one set of clothes for another, then headed for the Gulf of Mexico to meet up with Captain Mike Morehart. Mike and Ashley had been pirating together for years, sharing maps, buying, selling and trading various commodities, including large sums of money.

Mike had built the Manutea—a ninety-one-foot schooner with cargo hull, state of the art navigation and communications—to harness the wind. He was always searching for how best to serve and preserve the environment and improve man's understanding of the earth and her waters. He and his various crews had already sailed her around the world three times. This time Mike and Ashley had mapped out a Spanish galleon off the Gulf of Mexico they hoped to find and explore.

Two days into the journey, Mike's radio went out. He wasn't too concerned. Something always went dead. For centuries men had navigated by the constellations without communication and arrived safely to port. All I could think about was the Spanish galleon that didn't. Seasoned sailors seem to have an oversized confidence in their and their vessel's abilities to navigate any unforeseen storms. But Ashley trusted Mike and I trusted Ashley.

Rolling swells started on our third afternoon out. While the sensation of a moving car or the train over a long period of time worried me, this rolling—rock, sweep, dip—did not. It lulled me like the swing of a hammock. I made my way to the foredeck and sat facing the wind, embracing nature's incredible power. By late afternoon the roll had become waves and each set rolled in bigger than the last. Cramps and a dull but constant pain gripped my stomach. I vomited, then vomited again and again. On hands and knees, I crawled to the hatch and eased down the ladder below decks, latched the portholes. I had nothing left to vomit, yet the powerful cramps continued. Night fell and the intensity of the storm increased. From below deck I heard wind and waves lashing the rigging, Ashley and Mike yelled to each other as the wind ate their words. I reached for my pills.

Day broke calmer. By afternoon, we made landfall. I couldn't get off the Manutea fast enough and had already told Ashley I wasn't sailing back. He took it in stride as we ambled hand in hand down a wide stretch of white-sand beach. Perhaps it was the sleepless night that made him so amiable and accepting. Whatever it was, I was grateful not to have to plead my case as I had unsuccessfully on the train. In disagreements, I found it difficult to stand up to Ashley's assumed intellectual superiority. His retorts left me grasping at tiny, brittle straws of reason that even to me didn't quite hold together.

Walking in the shore-break with my white pant legs rolled up, I didn't notice the wet. I noticed the color. Red. A huge wash of it soaking my pants and turning the water around my shins scarlet. I hadn't even known I was pregnant. This was the second time we'd lost a baby. The first had been in July when we were deep into planning the wedding and building what would soon be our home on the lake at Crystal Island Ranch. I had noticed acute pains in my right ovary and received a diagnosis of pregnancy. I was shocked. We'd been trying to prevent pregnancy. However, it appeared a tiny soul had wanted to come through. Ashley and I were thrilled and told all our family.

Our euphoria was short-lived. Medication I'd been taking was potent and known to cross the blood-brain barrier. The doctors felt the baby would most certainly have brain damage. I was more than a month along and I'd been taking the medication the entire time. I was advised to terminate.

A crushing decision, first at nineteen, then at thirty-eight. The reasons differed, but the decisions haunted me nonetheless. At nineteen, my concern had been the impact of a pregnancy on my already emotionally overwrought parents in the wake of brother Bill's car wreck and new status as a quadriplegic. At thirty-eight, what unsettled me was the prospect of raising a handicapped child. How much brain damage? No one could answer. I could not burden my health or my marriage with a brain-damaged child.

We told family I'd lost the baby.

ESTANCIA RANQUILCO, NORTHERN PATAGONIA, ARGENTINA

DECEMBER 1987

AN HOUR'S FLIGHT FROM San Martin de los Andes in Ashley's little Cessna 172 tail-dragger brought us through the Cordillera to Ranquilco. Thirty minutes out, Ashley contacted his sister Annie via radio at the estancia to make sure several gauchos would meet us with horses and ox carts for the luggage. On approach, we flew down the canyon and over the big house, tucked onto the shelf of hillside overlooking the river. The stone house was castle-like with its turret and broad terrace.

Gauchos and their families through the years had been the backbone of Ranquilco. Many of our gauchos had been born and raised on this land and had rarely been off it. Most had never driven. Rarely had they watched television. Originally, a small schoolhouse served the gaucho's children as well as country people from surrounding remote ranches. It was a limited education, but it was something, and allowed families to stay together. When Ashley had bought Ranquilco, he closed the school. The families moved to town as school was now mandatory for all children and the gauchos left lived at the ranch and went to town—five-hours away by horse—on the weekends.

Christmas. Tidings of comfort and joy. The stone castle with its thick, exposed beams. Vaulted ceiling in the main dining and living room. Central fireplace big enough to roast a whole goat. The challenge of the turret's spiral staircase leading to bed after many wine-soaked dinners.

Perfect, except for one obstacle—Ashley's family. His son T.A., now fifteen, and sister Annie, had seemed to join forces to make my life as miserable as possible. Dossie was easy-going, but detached in a friendly sort of way, while Ashley was oblivious to it all. Initially, I thought my discomfort was due to the fact this lifestyle was all so new and different. Ashley's family had been coming to Ranquilco for several seasons, but after a few weeks rolled by with Christmas and its recycled wrapping paper, I knew there would be no softening or open arms. Being Ashley's new wife, I ascended to the role of Patrona. There can be only one and Annie let it be known she resented the demotion. Coupled with T.A.'s surly teenage demeanor, and compounded by my lack of Spanish, I was left frustrated and ineffective. By the New Year, even Ashley had noticed and flew us out of Ranquilco to peace at Lago Lolog.

LAGO LOLOG, SAN MARTIN DE LOS ANDES, ARGENTINA

JANUARY 1988

ASHLEY FLEW US TO SAN MARTIN. From there, we drove the limping four-wheel drive truck to town for supplies, enough to last two-weeks. At the dock at Lago Lolog, Ashley loaded the boat for the trip to the cottage.

At Christmas time, Ashley had gifted me the oasis of Lago Lolog. Aside from Crystal Island Ranch, it was a place of deep connection. Lago Lolog was close to 500 acres and an hour's drive to San Martin, yet untainted by civilization. At the land's heart, lay the lake or Lago and our mile-and-a-half of unobstructed lakefront. An old wood cottage, set at the edge of a forest of coyoway trees, akin to Live Oaks, bordered a stream that spilled into the lake. Built in the days before indoor plumbing and electricity, the cottage had a large fireplace for warmth and cooking.

Windows faced the lake, where on windy days I let myself be mesmerized by the constant movement of wind over water, of waves and tiny whitecaps. An exquisite path above the lake wound through the forest of coyoway trees to a pastured rise where the property's lone horse often grazed. Around the house, plum and apple trees, long gone wild, had been pruned and bore the first signs of fruit. Rangy lilacs had spent their blooms in spring. The previous year, Ashley had hired Hugo to reclaim the fruit trees and lilacs and to till the remnants of the abandoned garden and plant it anew. This fairytale landscape became my muse.

Ashley and I decided I would camp at Lago Lolog for two weeks. I had my art supplies and new Dalmatian puppy. The cottage's cat had just had kittens, and Hugo's garden was coming on—lettuce, carrots, beets, chard, onions, squash, tomatoes and herbs to season it all.

Hugo, who had helped build the big stone house at Ranquilco, was a talented man. He lived in San Martin with his wife and two children, and went to Lago Lolog as often as he could. He'd been responsible for lightly remodeling the cottage.

Once we unloaded, Ashley kissed me and motored the boat to other end of the lake. I was left with the horse. Two days in, the horse ran off. I was definitely stuck for two weeks. I gathered wood and learned the beauty of cooking by fire, living by candlelight, of bathing in water heated in the fireplace. It takes time to build and maintain a fire. Time to harvest the garden, wash and prepare food for cooking. Time to wash clothes in the stream, then hang them in trees to dry.

Time stopped. I bent to the rhythm of earth, fire, water, wind, with the sun and moon my timekeepers. I created some of my most beautiful pencil drawings—peas from the garden, the billy-goat skull that sat on the mantle, naked women dancing the fertility dance. I missed Ashley, but this time alone, away from his family, rejuvenated my spirit. The kittens, puppy and garden grew by the day. Rain and wind storms continually rolled over the lake. My biggest job was drying firewood. This time at Lago Lolog was heaven and I'd never felt better. The land had embraced me and I embraced it in a pioneering spirit that would heal me.

The natural lull of nature's rhythm started me thinking. To secure my place in the Carrithers' family hierarchy, I'd need to have a baby. I would love a child more than any other human, more than the animals I'd always turned to through the years when people had failed me. A soul was clearly trying to come through. My abortion at nineteen, the baby I'd had to terminate, and the miscarriage on the Manutea made that clear. I was quite sure the baby was a girl, so sure that I did a painting of myself and my three lost children. I vowed that if the creator would allow me to conceive once more, I'd dedicate my life to this being.

Ashley was due to fly in, yet the storms continued. Without instruments, small plane navigation in this sort of weather was dangerous. I remember sitting by the fire with the kittens and puppy and hearing the drone of the plane's engines. Ashley had said he'd make a pass over the lake to let me know he'd arrived and then motor out in the boat to get me.

The most dangerous times flying are take-off and landing. Likely it had been a sunny, windless morning at Ranquilco. It's only an hour flight to San Martin, however San Martin is often socked in and without instruments. We never knew leaving Ranquilco how the weather would be in San Martin. Sometimes we couldn't land. I willed the man I loved, the man I had chosen to father our child, to land safely. I surrounded him and his airplane in white light.

White light was a technique I'd been learning from the healers we frequently communed with in Aspen. Ashley had introduced me to the metaphysical world and I couldn't get enough of it. Healers, visionaries, channelers—so many different alternative medicines and ways of seeing the world and our relationship to it. After losing the two babies in Aspen, a healer had given me herbal tinctures sure to help strengthen my body for conception.

CRYSTAL ISLAND RANCH, COLORADO

MAY 1988

AFTER FINISHING OUT THE SUMMER at Ranquilco, our return to the northern hemisphere was a relief. Fortunately, by the time I'd returned to Ranquilco from Lago Lolog, T.A. had gone back to the states for school and Dossie with him, which left Ashley, Annie and me at the estancia. Annie and I gave each other a wide berth, made easier by a houseful of friends who'd flown down for two months of polo, wining and dining. Annie was big on keeping up appearances, so time with friends was festive. However, behind the scenes, especially in the kitchen, my minimal grasp of the estancia's needs and of Spanish often failed to get the job done. Annie was only too happy to help, lording it over me with a sly, self-righteous smirk. But I was past caring. I had more important things on my mind.

Back in my native land where groceries, medical care, and friends were within an hour's drive on paved roads, I settled in to our new home on the lake at Crystal Island Ranch. Our home was crafted from Crystal River rock, and logs harvested from the adjoining national forest with our Percheron draft horses. On our honeymoon, before our train out of Vancouver, British Columbia, we'd found the salvaged stained-glass windows and purchased them on the spot. We chose to keep the home simple. Recycled lake water plumbed into the kitchen, yes. Outhouse and bathhouse, yes. Electricity, no. Solar panels, yes. An outdoor wood-heated tub under the stars and mate pit, yes. Paved driveway, no.

Where I loved Lago Lolog's complete isolation and the cottage's ancient feel, the Patagonia winds often rendered the lake unusable—and I loved to swim. As much as I'd treasured my two weeks alone, I loved people and conversation too much to make it a permanent lifestyle. Crystal Island Ranch offered the same unparalleled natural beauty—the calm private lake spilling into streams that joined the Crystal River, the vista from Mate Hill of Mt. Sopris with the lake tucked against its base, and the river's path through the valley.

Near the house on Mate Hill, I held court daily with my newfound metaphysical friends and the horsey crowd; my animals if alone; or anyone who happened by. Yerba mate is a truth serum—give someone a mate and they spill their hearts. The ritual of mate and the herb itself, an herb that promotes mental alertness without caffeine, opened me to another dimension. The offering of mate to each person in the circle was parallel in hospitality and spirit to the offering of the peace pipe that I'd learned from Dik Darnell.

I developed my affinity for Yerba mate and the ceremony on one of my first trips to Ranquilco. Having driven an hour and a half from El Heucú to the summer grounds of Buta Mallin, where we were to saddle up and ride the two-and-a-half hours in, Ashley and I were greeted by gauchos around an open wood fire, sharing mate from a simple gourd. The *pave* or kettle was kept hot by the *cebador* or server, and the gourd, with its *bombilla* or straw, was passed from *cebador* to each person in the circle who, when finished, would pass it back to be refilled. And in this way time slowed and the fatigue and silence around the fire gave way to conversation. Our saddled horses idled under a massive shade tree with the cattle dogs stretched long near their feet as the heat of the day bled out and the evening's first cool breeze swept across the cordillera. After a final round for the stirrup, we mounted and rode.

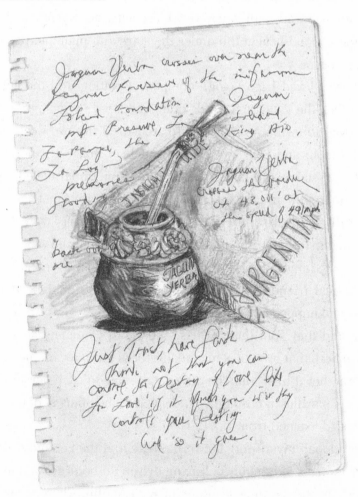

A SKETCH OF A GOURD-SHAPED YERBA MATE CUP,
ALONG WITH A FEW JOURNALED THOUGHTS. I DID
THIS ON A FLIGHT TO ARGENTINA.

Importing Yerba mate to Crystal Island Ranch was a natural extension of this new way of being in the world. A way that was unhurried and hospitable. Gathering kindling and wood and building the mate fire each morning carried forward the peace and tranquility I'd found at Lago Lolog where time had stopped. Once again, I bent to the rhythm of earth, fire, water, wind. Sun and moon time.

Moon time. My moon time had not come since October, since the miscarriage on the Manutea. On our return to Colorado, I knew I was pregnant. Knew when I'd conceived—at Ranquilco on a lazy summer afternoon in our bedroom in the stone house perched on a rock shelf overlooking the cordillera and the deep wet slash of the Rio Trocoman below. The time-worn song of river over rock, the wind bending the Lombardi poplars, and our desire the only sounds.

Given my complex medical history with MS, previous medications, and my age, thirty-nine by then, my obstetrician advised an amniocentesis to rule out any genetic defects or fetal abnormalities. None. Ashley and I rejoiced and spread the news. No more riding for me—I didn't want to chance losing this baby.

In the meantime, Ashley's sister Annie, who'd been so cold to me in Argentina, had come to live with us. Her heart had been broken and she needed a place to regroup and rebuild. Being an excellent cook and gardener, she took over those duties—a great relief to me, considering my macrobiotic diet.

Summer in the Rockies bloomed. Warm languid days, cool star-filled nights. The Fourth of July slipped by with our annual lake party with the rich and famous, the crazy and infamous. I spent many afternoons at the lake, floating on a surfboard, growing belly to the sun. Gentle waves and wind lulled me into a trance, as did the music of Dik Darnell. Dik was the adopted white grandson of Frank Fools Crow, the most important ceremonial chief in the Lakota Sioux nation. He had been the Lakota Sioux Medicine Carrier who presided at our wedding. Dik had founded the Etherean Music label and was an award-winning New Age musician. The drumming and flutes on his cuts produced a simultaneously earthy and earthly resonance, rocking my deepest soul. Dik introduced me to Native American ways—sweat lodges, healings, burning sage, the restorative gift of the peace pipe ceremony. I'd found a spiritual approach that fit.

Ashley and I had begun natural childbirth lessons. Also, couples therapy, on which he had insisted. Ashley was not happy with me pregnant. He felt trapped. Said he'd begun to realize on the train during the honeymoon that he'd married the wrong woman. Now he had a wife he'd actually have to support, rather than the other way around; a wife who wasn't a multi-millionaire with the power to buy his way in or out of pleasure or trouble; a wife with a disease he couldn't bother to learn about.

MILL POND PLANTATION
THOMASVILLE, GEORGIA

THANKSGIVING 1988

ASHLEY HAD SCHEDULED US TO GO to Argentina at the end of November via Sedg's Mill Pond Plantation. He wanted to be quail hunting by Thanksgiving. I wanted to stay home and get to know my daughter—Alixandra Sky. She'd arrived via cesarean on a snowy morning the second week of November. The cesarean had been advised to prevent any paralysis the trauma of delivery might incite. Given my age and history with MS, I couldn't risk a natural birth.

When the surgical nurse had handed me my daughter, I felt absolutely no connection and it scared me. This alien being I was now responsible for had a thatch of auburn-red hair and her nose and forehead seemed permanently creased. Ashley grinned ear-to-ear as our first family photo was snapped. Easy for him—he wasn't the one with tubes up his nose and his abdominal muscles sliced clean through. Luckily, my delivery hadn't induced any MS effects and our daughter was healthy. The only problem was I was so nervous my milk wouldn't let down. Her bleating cry during diaper changes put me in a panic that stopped my milk. I turned diaper duty over to Annie and Ashley.

We drove my VW camper van to Mill Pond because I insisted. I hadn't felt ready to fly two-and- a-half weeks after giving birth. Plus, after all the time Spot and I had spent traveling the country in it to raise money for The Race Against MS, the camper was a little piece of home. Ashley allowed me this eccentricity, but made it clear he thought it was absurd. When I'd packed my electric breast pump, Ashley took it right back out. "Not a chance, Ginny. Don't be ridiculous."

The saving grace of that Thanksgiving at Mill Pond Plantation was a black woman on staff who had nannied for years. I don't remember her name now, but will never forget her kindness and easy way with me and Sky as she helped me relax and learn the primal language of a mother's love.

SAN MARTIN DE LOS ANDES, ARGENTINA

DECEMBER 1988

A BABY. A DOG. A CRATE AND MASSES of luggage on the sidewalk outside the International Terminal in Buenos Aires. I stood in the sun in the middle of it all, shading baby Sky as Ashley negotiated us into several taxis and instructed them to take us to a used car dealer at the outskirts of the city. I wanted to fly. Get to San Martin as quickly and efficiently as possible. Still not fully healed from my cesarean, still having a bit of trouble nursing, and with a young dog in tow, a 1500 km drive across Argentina seemed too much.

I didn't understand Ashley's insistence on driving until he announced we'd be stopping in the Province of La Pampa to see Estancia La Guardia Vieja, a property he'd recently purchased sight unseen, unbeknownst to me, with money borrowed from his mother,

Dossie. I vividly remember him driving, Sky cradled in my left arm, asleep, and the sandwich in my right hand that somehow hit him square in the temple.

La Guardia Vieja, at 5000 acres, was to be Ashley's Mill Pond Plantation, complete with quail hunting. Ashley's childhood dream was to run parallel to Sedg in all things extravagant, which was totally unrealistic on largely impassible land, harboring trees with long piercing thorns and black spiders the size of small dinner plates. But most egregious was the water. It was salty. Too salty to use for anything without investing in an expensive filtration system. The house was in complete disrepair. More money from Dossie brought in potable water, quail, and a local family to care for them. Ashley had found a builder to remodel the house, but so far nothing had been done.

I was still very much in love with Ashley, in spite of his resistance to marriage and fatherhood, in spite of dragging us away from our safe haven of Crystal Island Ranch too soon after Sky's birth. I'd hoped time as a family would bring us closer, but our dependency seemed to drive him further from us. There was hardly ever a time that Sky and I were alone with him without his family or a group of friends or Sedg. Safety in numbers.

I was adamant about not immediately traveling to Ranquilco. Given that my cesarean hadn't yet fully healed and that Sky was only six-weeks old, San Martin seemed a wise place to rest and recoup for at least a few more months before heading into the backcountry. Ranquilco's nearest hospital was nine hours by horse. The flight took an hour, *if* the plane was in working order, *if* the weather cooperated. The estancia had a shortwave radio, but that was it as far as communication.

Ashley's solution was to buy a house ten-minutes outside of San Martin. The cement block house needed remodeling, but was on an exquisite piece of land. The road was good and the property much closer and safer than Lago Lolog. Here, I'd have everything I might need if something went wrong. My caution stemmed from my own childhood colic. My wheezing for air had been the cause of many emergency room visits and several close calls.

It took the better part of a week to settle in. Seeing I still needed help, Ashley hired a maid. The maid arrived the following day, along with Dossie and Annie, who were on their way to Ranquilco for the season. Within a few days of their departure, Ashley announced he, too, was leaving for Ranquilco. I wasn't ready. "You don't have to come," he gestured around the living room with a broad sweep of his arm. "You have a maid, a car, a house ten-minutes from town." He was yelling now. "What do you want from me?" In the entirety of our marriage, it was the biggest fight we'd ever have. He screamed, "What do you want from me?" over and over until he was hoarse. By morning, he'd lost his voice.

What does any new mother want from her husband? Companionship, love, kindness, caring. A family. So far, this trip had been a nightmare. In Colorado, he'd told me I didn't have to come to Argentina with Sky. That was the last thing I wanted to hear. Even though Ashley had never been one for intimate conversation, I'd thought the quality of his love for me was as complete and whole as mine for him. The last thing I wanted was to stay behind without him. I'd mistaken his generosity as a provider for the love and emotional security I'd always craved, security that had been absent in a childhood fraught with the minefields of physical and mental illness. Ashley wanted *his* family, the family he already knew and trusted, the family who'd loan him money and not impinge on his lifestyle.

In hindsight, I realized Ashley would never have married me had I not brought the gift of Dick Brunswick's money. Several months before we married, Ashley had asked me for $100,000 to pay off a debt on the middle house on the lower part of Crystal Island Ranch. He was hedging the loan on the future performance of South Wall Technologies. Ashley had started the solar window company with his ex-wife's co-signature. At one time, it looked like it would make

Ashley a very, very rich man. Lockheed Aerospace and 3M had been participating in product development for aerospace and defense capabilities. The company was about to go public. Ashley, being the majority shareholder, was given the option to sell his shares for a healthy profit. I suggested he sell enough to pay off the ranch's debt, but he refused, saying the stock would double or triple within a year. Not trusting the stock market, I voted for paying off the ranch, as I knew what it was worth, and would be worth in the future.

Since we weren't yet married and the ranch was in Ashley's name, not mine, I didn't give him the money.

ESTANCIA RANQUILCO, NORTHERN PATAGONIA, ARGENTINA

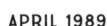

APRIL 1989

IN THE END, I LEFT THE MAID, the car, and the security of the house ten minutes from San Martin, and headed to Ranquilco with Ashley. Over that summer Sky and I both began to flourish. Sky fattened with my now free-flowing breast milk. We rode. Sky sat in front of me on the pellon, the double-thick sheepskin that gauchos use for a comfortable ride, and she'd drift off, snug against me. I appeared to be in nearly full remission. There were days, then weeks, that went by without me worrying about an activity's potential to instigate a relapse. The words Multiple Sclerosis slipped from my vocabulary, as did my fear of living well and fully.

The most valuable of Ashley's gifts was bringing me to this remote estancia in the middle of Northern Patagonia. I arrived in December a terrified new mother, but the simplicity of depending on the land for sustenance, inspiration, and clues to the passage of time rejuvenated me. Gravity-fed fresh spring water into the house, and wood-fire-heated river water to bathe. Spring water slipped through a stone cool-box to preserve perishables. We ate goat or sheep for most meals, as the meat kept for three days or more when hung in screened boxes. Steers were slaughtered for large parties that could consume the meat within two to three days. A lush organic garden provided greens, squash, fruits. Candles lit our evenings. Fires cooked our food. I started counting moons instead of months. I felt storms coming and reveled in the ever-changing Patagonia weather.

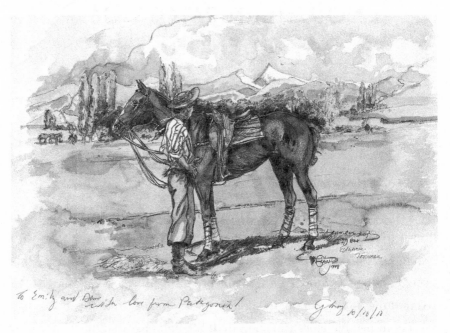

TITLED "PLAY PATAGONIA POLO", I PAINTED THIS WATERCOLOR WHILE IN JUNIN DE LOS ANDES, PATAGONIA, ARGENTINA IN 1998.

Estancia living was like living in your own small town. As I have never been comfortable in town, I made my own camp, Daughter of the Moon, named from the Lakota Sioux teachings.

Within walking distance of the casco, I could still fulfill my Patrona duties while honoring my need for sacred space. At Daughter of the Moon, I demanded respect for my privacy, which was imperative, as many have never learned or have forgotten how to honor the sacred space of others.

I brought south the teachings of Dik Darnell, Medicine Carrier of the Lakota Sioux. I sought sustenance from mother earth. I slept on her breast nearly every summer night for four-months at Daughter of the Moon. Sometimes with Ashley, and in the beginning, always with Sky. Ashley needed his sacred space too, and Daughter of the Moon was definitely a feminine place.

I co-created a beautiful spot. The gauchos built a stone arch entrance. Waterfalls cascaded over the far hillside. A reflection pond doubled the brilliance of the moon and at the center of it all was a fire pit for mate. For sleeping, I leveled out an area the dimension of a king-size bed with a big stone as headboard, then filled the bed with sand and slept on pellons with my sleeping bag and ponchos, and down pillow. My stallion, his broodmare, and their babies lived with me at Daughter of the Moon and would often visit in the night. First, I'd hear the vibration of their hooves, then the sound of leaves crunching and the soft snort as they exhaled over my head to say hello. This was my real home. I rarely slept in the suite in the big house.

Occasionally, I'd invite a few broadminded estancia guests to Daughter of the Moon for afternoon mate, but never in the morning, as that was my prayer time during which I prayed to the seven directions. In Native American tradition, as I'd learned from Dik Darnell, there are four directions—north, south, east, west. In developing my own spiritual tradition, I added above, below and within. After my morning mates, always sprinkled with different herbs from the land, Sky and I would join Ashley in his office at the casco for another mate while he gave the gauchos their daily work orders. Ashley would bounce Sky on his knee, then balance her as he reached for the *pava* on the fire to continue serving the mate.

Later in the morning, I'd often hike thirty-minutes to Temple Rock to do my morning pages— three longhand journal pages each day. Sometimes, I'd take friends and Sky to Temple Rock, the highest point above the estancia. The 360-degree view of the cordillera encompassed a great deal of the Trocoman River Valley and its steep-walled canyons. At sunset, I'd ride my stallion bareback. But never was I truly alone, because the pair of eagles that lived in the valley often soared close enough that I could see the light in their eyes. They were my totems, my power allies. Once again, I prayed to the seven directions.

For the rest of the summer we lived the life of wealthy, landed people. Flying to friends' estancias for polo, parties and overnights. A continuous stream of guests at our own estancia kept the atmosphere festive. One sweltering January morning, we flew to the estancia of one of Argentina's finest polo pony breeders to look at a few broodmares. Star-struck by the setup and a little drunk after a two-and-a-half-hour lunch, Ashley bought the lot of them, with a stallion to begin breeding our own stock. So there were horses to care for and the staff to manage, too, in addition to other responsibilities. Ashley handled the gauchos and volunteers, while five people worked with me to maintain the casco: Ashley's sister, Annie, who cooked and ran the garden; the gardener who helped her; Guzman, my personal gaucho; a nanny for Sky; and a full-time woman to wash, clean and bake bread. As Patrona, my biggest challenge was translating my instructions into Castellano to get the work done in a polite way. Ashley said I was nicer to the people who worked for me than I was to him. He managed people with an arrogant offhandedness I found embarrassing and abrasive. I'd always believed a little interest and kindness toward the people working with you day-to-day goes a long way in creating cooperation and harmony.

As the Lombardi poplars rained gold heart-shaped leaves and the morning cold lasted until midday, the meat bees began to come out in a quantity and ferocity I'd never seen. Meat bees can strip a carcass in an afternoon. They'll attack any open mouth for the next bite of meat or any exposed skin smelling of it. Crawling around in the grass, Sky was attacked enough times that I thought it time to return to Colorado. Ashley wasn't ready, so I took Sky and left.

CRYSTAL ISLAND RANCH, COLORADO

MAY 1989

OUR HOME, CRYSTAL ISLAND RANCH, was filled with baby things I'd collected during my pregnancy. The tiny toys and outfits, many of them already outgrown, made me wistful for that time before Sky, when it seemed life with Ashley could go nowhere but up. I remembered the therapy and brushing off his concerns, because I thought they would pass. Back then, I'd refused to see anything that might threaten my safety, security and joy. Now, back at Crystal Island Ranch with Sky, I realized I had more of a love affair with our new baby than I did with my husband.

Ashley extended his stay at Ranquilco and I was left wondering about the $100,000 debt on Crystal Island Ranch. As much as I'd loved my summer at Ranquilco, I began to understand that Ranquilco was *his* dream, while Crystal Island Ranch was mine. I figured the best way for us to pay off the ranch was to take part of 3000 acres and partition seven, twenty-five acre lots. I contacted the best real-estate lawyer in Aspen. Each lot would be worth $250,000. Given Ashley's passion for polo ponies and buying and selling airplanes and land, it seemed time to generate some cash rather than wait for South Wall Technologies to make him a billionaire.

Within a year, the stock had dropped to half its value, while the land's value continued to rise.

On his return to Colorado, Ashley confronted me about my intention to subdivide. He said he wanted nothing to do with it. "I'm not a land pimp."

Interesting, coming from the man who'd bought estancia La Guardia Vieja in La Pampa at the spur of the moment with money borrowed from his mother, then purchased the house close to San Martin with a car and the maid so he could leave me there and not be inconvenienced. And now, there were already murmurings about selling La Guardia Vieja as the quail weren't thriving because the expensive water filtration system was still not in. Also, the house needed more work than originally thought, but bless him, the airstrip and polo field were in.

I had to pay more attention to finances. Knowing we should have sold enough shares of South Wall Technologies to pay off the ranch, I said as much, but Ashley dismissed me. There would be no discussion or debate with him over what I thought might be a bad decision. As he had no respect for my opinion, it just didn't pay to confront him.

EL HEUCÚ, NORTHERN PATAGONIA, ARGENTINA

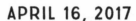

APRIL 16, 2017

WHERE DOES THIS STORY END? Where does any story end? Maybe it ends when I am fifty-two and triumphant in having survived the ravages of MS in spite of ignoring that therapist's advice to stop traveling and slow down. From 1987, when I met Ashley, through 2005, I migrated from the northern to southern hemisphere every six months. First following Ashley, then following Sky, then against all advice from family and friends, in 2005, I moved permanently to Argentina.

From 2005 through 2010, I summered in El Heucú and wintered in San Martin de los Andes or Cordoba, where the climates and company were near perfect.

Or maybe the story ends when, after ten years of marriage to Ashley, when I am in an Aspen attorney's office ready to sign papers for a legal separation because in his effort to keep financially afloat and feed his lust for land, polo ponies and planes, he has eviscerated the heart of our land holdings. Crystal Island Ranch is gone. Lago Lolog is gone. What remains is *his* dream of Ranquilco and lesser properties that he will eventually come to sell or leverage away. I am legally responsible for half of his debts and they are mounting. I need to protect our assets. I want financial security for Sky. At the time, she is only five. I also want a father, her father, for her and for me. The hell of it is, I still love Ashley despite his precarious financial risks. He is like a cat, somehow always managing to land on his feet.

It broke a piece of me to lose Crystal Island Ranch, *my* dream, and Lago Lolog. Both places were spiritual touchstones. But what cut deepest after five years of marriage was Ashley's proposition of an open marriage. He wanted me to remain his wife, and mother of daughter, Sky, and Patrona of Ranquilco, but he wanted to sleep with whomever he wanted, whenever he wanted.

At the conference table in the lawyer's office, my consciousness sits somewhere outside myself listening as the attorney explains why it would behoove me to divorce now rather than legally separate for two years. "It's going to happen eventually anyway," the attorney says assuredly, as if he has the crystal ball for which I've been searching all along. There are two sets of documents prepared. Somehow my pen inks the set that irrevocably severs the marriage. But not our link, because between us will always be daughter Sky.

Perhaps the story ends right after the divorce in 1997, when I am financially stable, but emotionally adrift. Dr. Dick, who'd promised to *always* be here for me, is dead. After being diagnosed with Rheumatoid Arthritis about the time Ashley and I married, he began to cut back on his surgeries. He stopped practicing medicine within a year of his diagnosis, unwilling to entrust the lives of his young patients to hands he had come to doubt.

In Salta, Argentina in 1993, I received a phone call from a friend saying Dick had committed suicide. He had shut himself and his Dalmatian, the son of my old dog Spot, in the Rolls Royce's garage and left the engine to run. When Norris, his cleaning lady, found him, she also found a check for $50,000 made out to her with a note, "Use this to educate your son."

I would like to think that in the end, Dick found love. During one of my visits north, he had introduced me to Mary, a Texas oil woman with whom he was in a relationship. They fit well together, seemingly happy and in love. Would you kill yourself if you were in love? I think not. Later, I heard they had parted ways prior to his suicide, but I don't know for sure. What I do know is that Dick died at age fifty-five, the same age my father took his life. Dick's death, like my father's, robbed me. In my father's time, then in Dick's, no matter how far I strayed, there had always been someone to watch over me, even if from afar.

The story could end with the call I receive from Sandra within a few months of Dick's death. I am back in Colorado, organizing a major, multi-media art show to promote Ashley's environmental organization, Island Foundation. Sandra says Mother is extremely ill and that I should come. How many times have I been called to Mother's death-bed and then she would not die? The show is in days. Susie goes to Chicago to be with Sandra and together, by phone, they keep me posted, moment to moment, until Mother quietly passes. Pearl Virginia Roberts Tice had died.

Virginia Pearl Tice Neary Carrithers did not go. Nor did I travel to Waterloo for the funeral, though I heard it was well attended. I heard the highlight of the eulogy was when Sandra told those gathered what Mother had said to her several years prior: "Sandra, we have to hurry up and spend this money before it's all gone." Even people at their craziest, can surprise you in their wisdom.

Another ending could be my major relapse of MS in 1993 following the deaths of Dick, Mother, and Ashley's intention to participate in an open marriage, whether or not I was willing. I begged him to be discrete. For Sky's sake, I begged. For Sky's sake, I moved us into my ancient VW Vanagon camper, parked at a friend's ranch near Aspen. I will never forget standing in my friend's driveway, holding Sky's hand, when Ashley and his new girlfriend rolled up in her top-down red convertible. He leapt out and, holding her hand, told Sky that they were off to Boulder for three or four days. Bile rose in my throat, choking back anything I may have said, but really, what could I have said to that?

Or maybe the story ends right here at the chacra in El Heucú. Always I fought to overcome MS. At thirty-six, had I accepted that therapist's advice to stop traveling and slow down, I'd have been dead *before* fifty-two, from atrophy and boredom if nothing else. Always I have stood beside my choices, taken what life has given me and made the best of it. I make no excuses for my own poor decisions, my impulsivity and living life large. When life corrects me via MS, or Messenger of Spirit as I came to call this dis-ease during my 1993 relapse, I listen.

At sixty-eight, my body has succumbed to the ravages of Multiple Sclerosis. I can no longer pretend that if I just work hard enough I will walk again. I am giving up the fight against disease. I will no longer take the pain pills that require another pill to prevent the shredding of my stomach lining. If I am in pain, I will go to bed. So what if I'm not up in my wheelchair half the day? I will keep doing my exercises five days a week because I feel better when I do them. I accept my staff as they are. I accept what attention Sky has to give and that I must now defer my need for her attention to the needs of my grandson, Leo. I accept two-year-old Leo's noise and boundless energy and rejoice in his willingness to climb into bed with me and watch silly cartoon clips Sandra sends via Skype.

Finally, I come back to the land, to the fall silhouettes of Lombardi poplars dancing gold and half-naked outside my bedroom window on these grey and gloomy days. Dried rose petals, lavender, comfrey and other herbs from the garden liven my morning and afternoon mates.

Mates are no longer taken outdoors over an open fire, but the memories of those fires, of Daughter of the Moon and Mate Hill and every other mate I've shared with stranger and friend alike, are offerings of the goodwill and peace I carry within me. This chacra is a grounding place, a healing place. A place to which my daughter will always return. This is the life she has chosen and because it is hers, it is mine as well. My paralysis is of the body and I accept my body as it is, while my spirit is free to soar.

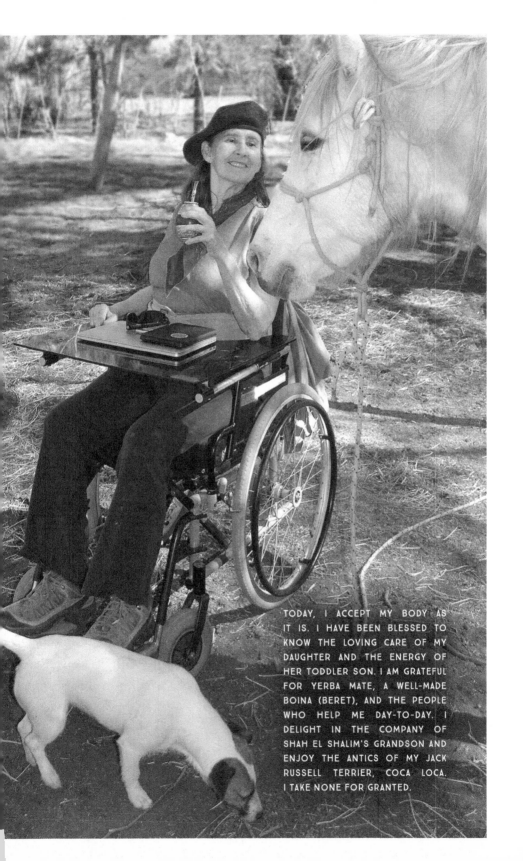

TODAY, I ACCEPT MY BODY AS IT IS. I HAVE BEEN BLESSED TO KNOW THE LOVING CARE OF MY DAUGHTER AND THE ENERGY OF HER TODDLER SON. I AM GRATEFUL FOR YERBA MATE, A WELL-MADE BOINA (BERET), AND THE PEOPLE WHO HELP ME DAY-TO-DAY. I DELIGHT IN THE COMPANY OF SHAH EL SHALIM'S GRANDSON AND ENJOY THE ANTICS OF MY JACK RUSSELL TERRIER, COCA LOCA. I TAKE NONE FOR GRANTED.

AFTERWORD

THE TIMELINES FOR THIS BOOK were drafted with various volunteers starting in 2009. Over the course of years since, I have come to have much respect and gratitude for the evolution in my relationships with Ashley, his son T.A., and his sister Annie. The harshness and hardness between us all since the years of the marriage and subsequent divorce has fallen away, replaced by a mutual respect, kindness, and concern for one another. Now that we've all grown, and with space and distance between us, it's as if we're all family again.

On I go, mostly happy, but mourn the loss of my drawing and painting hand. There are artists who paint with their brushes in their teeth or in their toes, but that is not me. I will continue to live one moment at a time with the peaceful presence I've come to cherish. May we all be blessed by the Great Creator.

With love to all.

Virginia Tice Neary Carrithers

EL HEUCÚ, NORTHERN PATAGONIA, ARGENTINA

APRIL 20, 2017

ACKNOWLEDGEMENTS

I AM SO BLESSED to have received so much help from so many people over the years. I can't acknowledge them all; you know who you are! Thank you, thank you from the deepest part of my heart.

I love you all.